THE
PERFECT FIT
DIET

THE PERFECT FIT DIET

Create your own weight-loss plan,
based on your tastes,
your genes and your lifestyle

Dr Lisa Sanders

RODALE

This edition first published in the UK in 2005 by
Rodale International Ltd
7–10 Chandos Street
London W1G 9AD
www.rodale.co.uk

Designed by Leanne Coppola/Abbate Design
Printed and bound in the UK by CPI Bath
using acid-free paper from sustainable sources.
1 3 5 7 9 8 6 4 2
A CIP record for this book is available from the British Library

ISBN 1–4050–7740–9

This paperback edition distributed to the book trade by Pan Macmillan Ltd

NOTICE
This book is intended as a reference volume only, not as a medical manual. The information given here is designed to help you make informed decisions about your health.
It is not intended as a substitute for any treatment that may have been prescribed by
your doctor. If you suspect that you have a medical problem, we urge you to seek
competent medical help.

Mention of specific companies, organizations or authorities in this book does not
imply endorsement by the publisher, nor does mention of specific companies, organizations or authorities in the book imply that they endorse it. Internet addresses and
telephone numbers given in this book were accurate at the time it went to press.

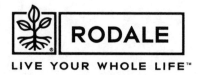

RODALE
LIVE YOUR WHOLE LIFE™

＊

For Tarpley and Yancey,
the best friends and daughters a mother could have.

CONTENTS

ACKNOWLEDGEMENTS

This book initially grew out of a research project I worked on with my friend and mentor, Dr Dawn Bravata. Her warmth, intelligence and discipline have been a model for me. Her faith in me and in this book never flagged, even when mine did.

I am also indebted to my sister Shelley, who shared with me the ups and downs of her personal struggle with her weight and let me share them in these pages. In addition, I could always count on my sisters Andrée and Leslie to help me keep my language and ideas tied to the world outside the doctor's office.

I am grateful to the patients who shared their stories with me. They have been my inspiration and education. If, as Montaigne says, experience is the test of medicine, their lives have been the textbooks, teachers and exams in my understanding of all that is in this book.

Josh Horwitz, of Living Planet Books, transformed my ideas into a book by believing in them and in me. Gail Ross, my agent, has been unstinting in her enthusiasm. My editor, Mary South, always brought a crisp, fresh perspective to this book. Her insights and skill made *The Perfect Fit Diet* a little closer to perfect. And the aptly named Amy Super always kept me organized – no small task. I'm grateful for the hard work and thoughtful insight of Jillian Stewart, who taught me about crisps and courgettes. Many, many thanks.

I must also thank Joel Lovell, Megan Liberman, Paul Tough, Ilena Silberman and Dan Zalewski, my editors at *The New York Times Magazine*. Their skilful editing taught me much of what I know about writing and everything that I know about writing well.

I owe thanks to Dr Julie Rosenbaum, my colleague at the Yale Primary Care Residency Program, and Valerie Duffy, a researcher and nutritionist at Yale School of Medicine and the University of Connecticut. Each brought a careful scientific eye to the manuscript, saving me from all manner of embarrassment; whatever errors remain are mine alone. The meal plans were developed with the help of a marvellous dietitian, Marcie Garcia.

Thanks also to Tony Horwitz, Geraldine Brooks and their dining room table, where so many ideas have been born. Dr Anjali Jain provided me with an important sounding board for many of my ideas. Margaret Spillaine and Bruce Shapiro were ever ready to supply advice and comfort, as needed.

Steve Huot, the director of the Yale Primary Care Residency Program, encouraged my interest in obesity from its start and remains an essential support. Thanks also to the staff of the Family Health Center: Dr. Henry Gift, Cindy Collette and June Detlefsen. Their humour and balance continues to make going to work a pleasure. Ideas always need a stimulating environment in which to grow. My tiny plot has been generously enriched by many scientists, researchers and friends who helped me bring this book to fruition. My thanks to Dr Gretchen Berland; Dr Laura Whitman; Dr Eric Holmboe; Dr Linda Bartoshuk; Dr James G. Gibbs; Kelly Brownell, PhD; Dr Walter Kernan; and Dr Patrick O'Connor.

Thanks also to the friends who made this book possible in ways too many to be recounted: Lindsay Patterson, Jenny Brown, Ian Ayres, Louise DeCarrone, Neale and Steve Berkowitz. Also, Juanita Stallings, Terry Lavallee, Mark Gracia, Joe Gallagher, Lea Bowman, Janel Hackney, Hiram 'Pat' Patterson and Martha Love. You are the heart and soul of this book.

But finally, it is Jack to whom I owe this book. His wisdom, insight, intelligence, wit and thoughtfulness shaped every idea, every page I have ever written. His love and devotion supported me from television, through medical school and residency and finally to my work as a physician and writer. His kindness and empathy, his humour and his incredible skills as an editor have enriched my life, my work and, of course, this book.

PART

THE NEW SCIENCE
OF WEIGHT LOSS

'TELL ME WHAT YOU EAT, and I will tell you who you are.'

That was the challenge delivered by Jean Anthelme Brillat-Savarin just over 200 years ago in his witty and insightful seven-volume masterwork on eating, *The Physiology of Taste*.

That quote has come down to us as, 'You are what you eat', a warning that what you eat will shape – quite literally – what you become. I would argue that the reverse is also true: who you are dictates what you eat in a fundamental way. What you eat is a direct reflection of who you are – genetically, culturally, psychologically and environmentally.

So, to rephrase Brillat-Savarin: 'You eat what you are'. If that is true, then the best diet for health and weight loss is going to be different for each of us. That's the premise of the Perfect Fit Diet.

1 CHAPTER

THERE IS A
PERFECT FIT DIET
FOR EVERYONE

WE LIKE TO THINK that behaviour as fundamental as choosing what we put in our mouths is well within the domain of human willpower – especially with the abundance and variety of foods available to us today. We can eat fruits and vegetables out of season, fish caught halfway around the world, and drink wine from grapes grown on every continent. But there is also an aspect to what we eat that seems beyond our complete control.

We may exercise our mighty wills in choosing where, what and when to eat, but we make those choices within a personal framework that is beyond choice. What foods we like or dislike, how we prepare them, why we want to eat in the first place, and why we feel full and satisfied at the end of a meal – all these aspects of eating are defined by our genetics, our culture and our lifestyle. We rarely ever think about them, yet they undoubtedly shape the world of eating within which we make our choices. These aspects cannot simply be willpowered into conformity with a list of healthy-eating principles.

In order to exercise real choice, we need to recognize the framework in our own lives that shapes and defines those decisions. This is something we know and accept in most parts of our lives – we rarely waste our time and effort in 'choosing' to make time stand still or the sun not set. We recognize that our choices must be made within the structure of a 24-hour day divided roughly in half to give us day and night.

Few things in the human experience are quite as unyielding to choice as time and the movement of the earth in its orbit. Yet, on the human scale, changing genes, culture, even lifestyle may be just as difficult to do. Recognizing the framework in which our individual choices are made is key to making changes that work. Science is beginning to show us and define many of the aspects that shape our choices – how our genes, our upbringing and our lifestyle create the structure in which our choices about diet are made.

This book is dedicated to helping you figure out your personal best diet by combining what science is learning about diet and weight loss with what you know about yourself. It takes both – the knowledge of medical science and self-knowledge – to bring about real change.

Modifying behaviour is hard. It's why so many of our New Year's resolutions are long forgotten by Valentine's Day, and why so many diets fail within days of beginning. Eating is a behaviour as complex and innate as any bodily function. And like all other aspects of human behaviour, change has to start with who *you* are and what *you* do now.

How many times has this happened to you? You meet a friend you haven't seen in a while and she looks great! You gently enquire, and she nearly explodes with the answer: after years of trying one diet or the other, she has finally found the right one. It was there the whole time and, now that she's on it, she can't imagine why she didn't see it before. It's so great, she says, and she gets to eat so many foods that she loves. She's never hungry, and she's losing weight like crazy. Before you know it, you're on the same diet too.

Once you're on it, however, it doesn't seem so great. These are not foods you want to eat. This is not the way you want to feel. You're not losing weight, just patience. You wonder what she was doing that you're not, why she feels so good and you don't. What's wrong with you?

There is nothing wrong with you, and there is nothing necessarily wrong with that diet. Why this is true represents a major shift in the way science is approaching all medicine and the issue of weight loss in particular: each of us is different from the other. What we're discovering is that not every treatment has the same effect on every patient. With weight control, that means that the regime that works for one person may not work for another. In diets, as in so many things, one size does not fit all.

Unfortunately, when a doctor sees a patient who wants to lose weight, he doesn't usually ask, 'What do you eat?' In fact, research suggests that he's much more likely to tell you what you *should* eat. It's the same diet he puts everyone on. He assumes, as so many of us have in the past, that for this one problem – being overweight – there is one cure, the diet he happens to prefer. And if you can't eat that way, then as far as your doctor is concerned, you're *choosing* not to lose weight. You clearly are just not motivated enough.

Or maybe he just tells you to eat less and exercise more. Chances are you would eat less, if you knew how. After all, you're probably the one who brought up the issue of weight loss in the first place.

This book is for people who know they are motivated enough but recognize that there are aspects of their eating habits that they can't seem to change. This book is for people who have tried to 'eat less and exercise more' but can't figure out how to do it without feeling hungry, irritable and tired. It's for people who want to eat in a sane and rational way that will make them feel good and be healthy while they lose weight. This book is for people who instinctively know that the claim of a magic bullet – the diet that works for everyone – is a myth, but they don't know how to figure out which diet will fit them.

There is a truckload of science out there about diets – much of it from new and exciting research – investigating what we eat, why we eat it, what makes us full and what makes us different from each other when it comes to diet. I've spent the past several years delving into the scientific literature, sorting through the good research and the not-so-good, looking for connections and hidden truths. The most compelling conclusion I've reached is this: the deeper you dive into the science of weight loss, the more the solution returns to the medical, psychological and lifestyle profile of each individual dieter. This book is designed to help you choose and customize a diet that fits you to a T – a diet that's a perfect fit because it's designed for you, and by you.

WHY I CREATED THE PERFECT FIT DIET

My education in the trials of weight management began years before I went to medical school. For decades I'd watched the collateral damage of failed dieting strategies at home, where my own family offered a telling example of the individual, and often elusive, nature of weight gain and loss.

My father's side of the family is overweight. My mother's side is thin. Unfairly, my wonderful older sister, Shelley, inherited my father's genes. Ever since childhood I've watched Shelley struggle with her weight. She's the classic yo-yo dieter. She goes on a diet, loses weight, falls off the wagon and, in a fit of despair, gains it all back. Over the years, she's tried every weight-loss fad on the market, as well as ones that weren't (such as amphetamines, when she was much younger).

Every failure is accompanied by a cycle of self-loathing and depression – which begins its own cycle of eating and exercise lapse. I love my sister, and it's painful to watch this intelligent and self-aware woman struggle to manage her weight. She remains locked in confusion – in part because the emotional issues involved are so threatening and, in part, because the facts about successful weight loss simply haven't been available.

Shelley is typical of the failed dieters I meet every day in my clinical practice. They see their lapses as moral failures, proof of their weak wills. But dieting isn't about moral strength – it's about compatibility between an individual and the chosen diet.

I'm writing this book to offer people like Shelley a way out of their cycle of guilt and shame by helping them find a weight-loss programme they can live with. They need hard information – so many dieting 'facts' are, in fact, fictions – and they need encouragement in tackling the very tough challenge of shedding weight in an environment rigged to make us gain.

This is a book for everyone who's struggled to lose weight, whether it's 5kg or 50 – it's for stressed-out, overweight executives; fat senior citizens; obese diabetics; potbellied middle-age labourers; chunky teenage girls; and every other variety of diet refugee you can think of.

My girlfriends, my patients and anyone I meet who finds out that I'm a 'diet doc' ask me the same question: Is there anything that actually works? These people have been beaten, both physically and psychologically, by a series of failed attempts at dieting. They are all looking for authoritative news about how to end the cycle of failed diets and finally succeed at weight control.

I'm convinced that this book, and the research it's based on, will be at the forefront of a new trend in personally tailored, medically based diets, as opposed to the one-size-fits-all approaches that have dominated the field for decades. Now that mainstream science is finally engaging nutrition and obesity as a serious field, we will be seeing more and more authoritative information about how our genes, our lifestyle and our personal taste preferences affect our ability to control our weight.

The Perfect Fit Diet is every dieter's long-sought compass for navigating the thicket of competing diet claims, the rational path for the thinking person who wants to lose weight.

A NEW LOOK AT WEIGHT LOSS

For the past several years, I've been working with a team of researchers at Yale and Stanford Universities. We've conducted a systematic analysis of hundreds of weight-loss studies dating back to the turn of the last century. Initially, we were looking at whether low-carbohydrate diets, such as the Atkins diet, were any better or worse than other types of diets. That study was published in the *Journal of the American Medical Association* (*JAMA*) in 2003. Now we're looking at the drugs used in dieting. In the course of my research, I have read literally hundreds of studies on the effect of different diets on weight loss and other aspects of health. After years of sifting through these studies, I was struck by a surprising pattern that seemed to defy conventional medical wisdom: all these diets did work – for some people.

Time after time, a study would show that a diet worked rather dramatically for, say, 10, 20, even 30 per cent of the people who tried it. How is it that nearly every good diet had winners and losers? Each seemed to have a cadre of people for whom the diet worked wonders, while other dieters failed miserably.

I became intrigued by the possibility that there was no single diet that worked for everyone but, rather, different diets that worked for different people.

Perhaps the key to weight loss was not the single best diet, or the most motivated person who was trying to lose weight – though clearly, diet and motivation are important. Perhaps the key lies in matching the right dieter to the right diet.

One of the conclusions of my research, and the research of many who came before, is that there are aspects of any diet that help predict how well it will work. For example, the lower the calorie content of the diet, the faster you will lose weight. And the longer the diet lasts, the more weight you will lose. But I realized that the key to eating fewer calories and staying on that diet depends on which diet and which individual.

This realization led me down a new path of inquiry: how could we use what we now know about weight loss to do for dieting what is already being done in other areas of medicine? More specifically: what list of questions would let you figure out which diet will work best for you? The search for that questionnaire was the genesis of the Perfect Fit Diet.

For a year, I worked to distill my research findings and extrapolate my clinical experience in treating overweight patients into a comprehensive questionnaire that anyone could complete. The questions range from straightforward information such as age, gender, weight and medical and family history, to detailed questions about lifestyle, eating habits and dieting history.

Once you've completed and scored your self-test, you'll be able to choose a weight-loss diet that best fits you and then further customize it based on specific aspects of how you eat, how you live and how your body works. The Perfect Fit Questionnaire takes an hour or so to complete, but the results will save *years* of searching for the right diet.

The Perfect Fit Questionnaire will:

- Identify which of the three basic types of diets will work best for you.
- Customize that diet to your medical, personal and family history, as well as your food preferences – creating an individualized diet that will appeal to your tastebuds and help you lose weight and achieve optimal fitness and health.
- Prescribe a diet and lifestyle plan that you can live with, happily, for the rest of your life.

The Perfect Fit Questionnaire is a direct translation of the doctor-patient Q&A I've been using to design personalized weight-loss plans for my patients. The answers to this questionnaire will empower aspiring dieters – whether obese or merely overweight – to successfully lose weight and keep it off, despite previous failed attempts.

WHY TASTE MATTERS

The Perfect Fit Diet is a customized dieting strategy built around your life and your preferences. In recent research, food preference has emerged as a key factor in satisfying hunger, and thus, in dieting success. (Nutritionists who work with people with diabetes have led the way in recognizing the importance of structuring a diet that works with a dieter's individual tastes.)

The Perfect Fit Questionnaire systematically uncovers what makes you eat, what tastes good to you, what relieves your cravings and what makes you feel satisfied. It incorporates that information into a personalized diet plan that will let you lose weight and maintain your ideal weight – because it's a satisfying eating plan that's a perfect fit for your lifestyle, your food preferences, your satisfaction – in short, a perfect fit for you.

Doctors, and just about everyone else, have thought of food preference as something trained and therefore malleable. If you wanted to lose weight, you would learn to love broccoli. If you couldn't, then you weren't serious about weight loss. Science is beginning to show us how little of food preference is really learned behaviour and how much is in our genes.

Recent research here at Yale reveals that what we think of as food preference or taste is actually a complex variety of factors, both genetic and acquired, physical and emotional. One of the most interesting findings is that some foods taste very different from one person to another, and that this sensibility exists on a genetic level. For example, some people have tastebuds that are keenly sensitive to even a trace of bitterness, and to them, vegetables like broccoli and Brussels sprouts and fruits like grapefruit can be extremely unpalatable.

In experiments, researchers have used a chemical called 6-n-propylthiouracil, or PROP for short, to test for this trait. Some people can detect even a trace of this chemical, while others cannot taste it at all. And it runs in families. If one of your parents has the ability to taste PROP, there's a good chance that you will have it too.

Researchers at the American National Institutes of Health recently identified a gene, called TAS2R, on chromosome 7. There are five forms of this gene, and which one you inherit determines whether you can even detect this bitter taste or to what degree you are sensitive to it. If you inherit a high degree of sensitivity to PROP from both parents, you will be able to taste even the tiniest amount of it. If you can taste PROP, then you may not be able to enjoy broccoli, because it simply tastes bitter to you. This means that hating vegetables may not be so much a moral failing as it is a genetic trait, like hair colour or the presence of freckles.

That's just one reason why accommodating individual food preferences is so important to a successful diet. My research, and that of others, shows that the primary predictor of a dieter's success is longevity: the longer you can stay on your diet, the more weight you'll take off and keep off. Deprivation diets only work in the short term; you can only stay on a diet that satisfies your fundamental food cravings. Unless your diet reflects your individual food preferences, it can't be sustained – because it won't be satisfying. The Perfect Fit Diet is the first weight-loss programme that respects this immutable law of human nature.

The bottom line of the new science of dieting is clear: if you can customize a diet to reflect your individual profile – your genes, your metabolism, your lifestyle and your food preferences – you can stay satisfied, and stay on your diet.

That's how you lose weight, and that's what this book is all about.

CHAPTER 2

WHY ONE SIZE
DOESN'T FIT ALL

THE IDEA BEHIND THE PERFECT FIT DIET should come as no surprise
to doctors. We already know that when it comes to treating disease,
one size does not fit all. Over the past 20 years, science has made dramatic discoveries in the areas of genetics and physiology, in the way
even the smallest cells in the body interact with different medications
and other therapies. Using this ever-expanding knowledge base, doctors hope some day to be able to devise an individualized treatment
regime based on a patient's medical profile, family history and what
we know about their genetics to control chronic diseases.

Take high blood pressure, for example. In just the past 20 years,
doctors have enjoyed the ability to prescribe several drugs that work
very well at lowering high blood pressure. Only recently, though,
have studies confirmed what doctors sort of knew in their gut: these

medicines have different effects on different people. In 1993, *The New England Journal of Medicine* published a study that compared the effects of six classes of high blood pressure medicines on a group of tens of thousands of former soldiers. Half the sample were white; half were black. This study supported what had been shown in several smaller studies – that blacks responded better than whites to a class of medicines known as calcium channel blockers and worse than whites to another class of medicines known as ACE inhibitors. Why that should be the case is still being investigated. That it is true has been accepted and shapes medical decision making thousands, perhaps millions, of times a day.

More recently, science has witnessed the birth of an entire field, known as pharmacogenetics, dedicated to the investigation of the inherited mechanisms that determine the responses to medicines that are used to treat everything from depression to cancer. This discipline grew from the widespread recognition that different patients respond differently to the same medications. For example, it has long been known that, while codeine is a wonderful pain reliever for most of us, for about 6 per cent of the population it offers no relief, no benefit.

It just doesn't work. Why? Because in order to work as a painkiller, codeine has to be broken down into its morphine base. Six to 7 per cent of the population is born without the machinery to perform this chemical transformation. This tiny genetic difference has no other effect except to make a good painkiller ineffective.

Here's another example, perhaps a little closer to home. Researchers in Canada wanted to see if obesity had a genetic component in addition to the environmental aspect already well-recognized. They found a group of twins and for several weeks fed these people 1,000 calories more than they normally ate. Each of the identical twins gained about the same amount of weight. Different twin sets, however, gained very different amounts – ranging from 4.5 to

18kg (10 to 40lb), proving that your genes strongly influence how you gain weight. Same 'therapy' (overeating by 1,000 calories a day) – very different results.

The same is turning out to be true for the treatment of obesity as well. For example, there is a segment of the population that processes carbohydrates differently from most of us. These people are born with a tendency to become resistant to the effects of insulin. Because of that difference, when they eat a diet low in fat and high in carbo-hydrates – a diet designed to lower cholesterol – they develop high cholesterol instead. Thus, the most popular diet among doctors and dietitians today is not the healthiest diet for those with this abnor-mality known as metabolic syndrome. Again, the same therapy will cause a very different effect in some of us.

It is likely that there are other differences between people and the way they process certain foods. For instance, there is good evi-dence that small dissimilarities in several genes make dramatic dif-ferences in the ways some people respond to the amount and type of fat in their diets. These mechanisms are still not well understood but are the target of much investigation right now.

There are variations not only in the way we process food but also in what causes us to feel full and stop eating. What makes us stop eating is actually a very complicated process and is probably con-trolled in many ways. However, it seems clear that when it comes to feeling that we've 'had enough', different people respond to different cues. We humans (as well as other species) have what is called sen-sory-specific satiety. What that means is that the enjoyment of any given flavour or texture begins to decrease as more of that food is eaten. But that can happen even while the appetite for other flavours or textures remains unabated. This is why we can feel full after a big meal of meat and potatoes and still find room for dessert. The appetite for sweets was untouched by the meal, and while you may or may not crave them, the sight or thought of them will appeal to your mouth even if your stomach is 'full'. This is thought to be part of the biological drive that encourages us to eat a variety of foods. Genetically speaking, this trait comes in handy on the savannahs of Africa if you're an Australopithecus primate trying to evolve into a human being. If you're plopped down in front of the TV, this trait has a whole other impact.

This form of feeling satisfied actually takes place in the mouth. We know this because researchers have done experiments where a food was eaten but wasn't allowed to reach the stomach. Research subjects were instructed to treat test foods the way an oenophile might treat wines at a tasting. They were to put the food in their mouths, savour it, then spit it out. The satiety for the flavour remained, even if the eater wasn't any more full.

Other research shows that volume of food is an important cue of satiety. In one experiment, 20 young men were given four different drinks before four meals. The drinks had the same total number of calories contained in different amounts of fluid. They drank this before eating lunch, and then the amount that each of the men ate at lunch was carefully monitored. The more fluid the men drank, the less they ate at lunch, even though the amount of calories in the drinks were the same. So volume of food is an important factor for many people.

Another powerful satiety cue for many people is the richness of a food – that is, how much fat and protein it contains. These foods trigger the release of specific digestive enzymes that not only work to break down these foods but also travel to the brain to report that you have eaten them.

It seems clear that different people have different responses to these various satiety cues. Two studies recently published in *The New England Journal of Medicine* identified a genetic variant in a small percentage of obese children, which made them produce less of a brain hormone known to cause a feeling of fullness. The clear implication is that these children may be obese simply because they never really feel full or satisfied by a meal. And there is evidence that, particularly in the overweight and obese, cues to stop eating can be overwhelmed by other feelings and sensations. So it may well be that once you start gaining weight, it becomes easier to gain more, because the body's usual mechanisms for controlling diet are misfiring.

Obviously, if you are trying to reduce the amount of food you eat, then choosing foods that will provide you with the loudest and clearest cues that you've had enough will be an important way to start any good diet. Forcing you to eat foods that don't relay this key signal to the brain – regardless of how good they may be for you – is going to be frustrating and undermine the 'willpower' of the dieter.

When you are selecting a diet, you will want one that gives you every possible advantage in staying on it: one that allows you to eat the foods you like and avoid the foods you don't like; one that takes advantage of whichever form of satiety speaks to your body best; one that is best for your body and your health. Can we predict who can stay on a diet and who can't? Anyone who has tried to diet knows that it's not about motivation. The key to being able to stay on a diet is how well that diet fits you as an individual.

YOU'RE ON YOUR OWN

Think about that feeling you have in the supermarket. You are pushing your trolley down the aisle. Products scream out to you from the shelf, by colour, by name, by packaging – they shout, 'BUY ME'. And it's hard to resist. The choice is intentionally overwhelming. The possibilities of what you could eat are almost endless. And who is in the supermarket making these decisions? Often, just you. All by yourself.

This, it should be said, is pretty new.

For most of the history of the species, there was something else accompanying any person who was trying to make the decision about what to eat. It was called culture. If you were Italian, for example, there was this whole tradition of eating called Italian food. The same was true regardless of where you came from: culture defined diet. There were cuisines – Sephardic Jewish, Irish, Hopi, French, Hawaiian, German, Chinese, Inuit, Scottish, Mexican. Cultural menus were largely inherited. And what were they? They were the passed-down wisdom of a people about what was good, healthy and available to eat in a particular place. This was what culture did. It set the framework for your diet.

Today, your cultural tradition is no match for the supermarket, where increasingly, one is able to assemble the essentials of every world cuisine. Market forces have overwhelmed culture. What that means is that we must all create our own private cuisine – an individual culture, as it were, that's just about you and all the choice that's out there.

The power of supermarket choice cannot be overemphasized. One of the lost stories about the fall of communism locates the precise moment when the wall started to crumble: it was in a Western supermarket. The story is told by Vassily Aksyonov, a Russian poet who had fled his homeland. He recalled a time in the late 1970s when the Soviet Minister of Agriculture was visiting Canada. The hosting officials took the Soviet bureaucrat to a supermarket. He walked up and down the aisles in stunned disbelief. How could this be? How could anyone have this much choice, this much food, just sitting on a shelf waiting to be bought? He noticed the aisles filled with people leisurely walking about, plucking one thing or another from the shelves, and came to the conclusion that the entire store was a setup. He was convinced that the supermarket was a 'Potemkin Village', a fake set filled with all these goods and a cast of actors playing the roles of consumers. And why? Just to make the Soviet visitor feel bad. He thought about life back home and how the average family bartered and bargained to get a simple staple like a tomato or a turnip. This display was just absurd in its excess. Really, he concluded, the Westerners had practically made fools of themselves with this obviously phoney store.

After the tour, the minister got back into his limo and headed toward another meeting with officials. On the way, they happened to pass another supermarket. The minister ordered the cars to stop. Smiling slyly, he said he would like to visit a supermarket not officially scheduled for the tour. So they parked, and apparently the first crack sending a fissure up the wall of communism occurred when that minister – a man named Mikhail Gorbachev – stepped through the automatic doors and saw the same scene he'd observed at the last store – the unreal amount of choice, the customers wandering the aisles.

It's hard for us to imagine just how peculiar supermarkets are in the history of humankind. They were invented after the Second World War and represented a sharp turn in the history of eating. For the first time in the history of food, each of us can choose almost anything on the planet to eat. The market has done what it does at its best: provide choice. Now we are swimming in it, and there is nothing between each one of us and the mountain of food out there except the way we as individuals decide to eat.

'I'M GOING ON A DIET!'

People say things like, 'Hey, I'm on a diet', or 'I'm going on a diet'. Doctors don't talk this way (or they shouldn't) because they know that we're all on diets, because a diet is simply what you eat. And that diet either works for you – lets you feel good and maintain a weight that also feels good – or it doesn't.

There are two aspects of traditional weight-loss dieting that bear commenting on. First, when you diet, you actually think about what you are going to eat and try to take control of that activity. This is the positive aspect of dieting.

Let's compare that to what happens under normal circumstances, when habit and the vast commercial forces determine what you eat. Most of us eat out of the home at least one meal a day – often even more – and if you haven't prepared yourself a packed lunch, the food choices we have to make are limited by what's available where we are when we need to eat. William Shakespeare said, 'There's small choice in rotten apples'. Yet that's the type of choice we have far too often when we have to eat away from home.

We know that, and so when we are dieting we know to plan ahead so that we don't have to either eat what's there or not eat at all. Planning what we eat is something we should do all the time, even when we are not trying to lose weight.

Here's what I think the downside of dieting is: we think of it as a temporary aberration, a deviation from our normal way of eating. This second assumption is what leads to so much of what is wrong with the whole culture of dieting.

Firstly, if we accept the idea that a diet is temporary, then any diet can be tolerated if it isn't for long. That's why it doesn't matter if the foods on the diet are the foods you like to eat – it's just temporary, until you lose the weight – and then you can go back to the old ways once again. In fact, in some ways, from this perspective, it's *better* if you don't like the foods. If you don't like them – goes this argument – you won't eat as much and you will lose the weight even faster. But that's a fallacy and it's why many diets don't work at all.

Secondly, if you think of a diet as temporary and different from the way you normally eat, a weight-loss diet allows you to avoid thinking about some of the ways that your *real* diet contributes to your difficulties in managing your weight. A weight-loss diet cannot teach you anything about the way you normally eat. A rotation diet or one that emphasizes only one food, which causes weight loss by severely restricting choice, has nothing to offer in a world where choice is practically limitless. It's just not realistic.

Albert Einstein once defined insanity as asking the same question over and over and each time expecting a different answer. If that is true, we are a society of nuts. We go on weight-loss diets to get rid of the weight our 'real diets' have put on us. Then, whether we are successful in our weight-loss diet or not, we go back to our old diet and, what do you know, if it made us gain weight before, it will do so again, because nothing has happened to change that diet.

In order to change what your diet does, you have to change your diet. If you just have a fling with some new and different weight-loss programme, you may or may not lose weight, but you probably won't stay on that programme forever. *You have to change the way you eat every day.* And that is not easy. (I don't have to tell you that. If you are reading this book, you are probably all too familiar with the difficulty of changing basic behaviour.)

So, how can we change such fundamental behaviour? I would argue that you have to work with what you have and try to shape that basic template into a diet that will work for you.

Over these next chapters, I will take you through the techniques that will help you design *your* perfect diet. You will learn to identify the foods you love and can't live without. Then you will learn how to put them together to create a diet that is both satisfying and good for you. You will learn what your eating triggers are and how to avoid them. You will learn how you respond to stress and how to keep that from ruining an otherwise perfect diet. Finally, you will figure out how to increase the activity level in your life to reduce stress and help you achieve and maintain your ideal weight.

I can't promise you it will be easy, but you already know that changing the way you eat is a tall order. What I can promise is that the best way to create a diet that works for you is by combining what you know about yourself with what we now know about dieting.

CHAPTER 3

HOW THE
PERFECT FIT
DIET WORKS

THERE ARE LOTS OF DIFFERENT WEIGHT-LOSS DIETS out there that work for different people. So how do you span the distance between you and your Perfect Fit Diet?

It's a customizing process that I sometimes compare to tailoring a suit. First, you need to find the basic pattern that fits your style; then you tailor the suit to your particular figure; finally, you accessorize to make it a perfect fit for your personal tastes and lifestyle.

Over the course of this book, I'm going to take you through the steps you need to take to create your Perfect Fit Diet.

- Step 1: Keep a 1-week eating and exercise diary.
- Step 2: Fill out the Perfect Fit Questionnaire.
- Step 3: Score the questionnaire to identify which of the three basic diet types is right for you: the Counting Carbohydrates Diet, the Counting Calories Diet or the Counting Fats Diet.
- Step 4: Customize that diet based on your food preferences and family medical history.
- Step 5: Customize your diet to fit your lifestyle – exercise, eating patterns, family and work life – to create an eating and exercise plan that fits your long-term weight goals.

STEP 1: THE 1-WEEK EATING AND EXERCISE DIARY

First, you will need to keep an eating diary for 1 week, writing down everything you eat or drink over the course of those 7 days. From a doctor's perspective, this is the equivalent of taking a patient history. You need to know in great detail precisely how, what and why you eat. This eating diary is the most important part of the information that you'll need to collect in order to fill out the Perfect Fit Questionnaire correctly.

During the week that you are keeping the eating diary, you may find yourself wondering, 'Should I put that in the diary?' The answer will always be yes. No matter what it is, if it went into your mouth and you swallowed it, write it down.

This goes for drinks as well. Even water. Write everything down. Everything. Trust me, the difference between what you think you eat and what you actually eat and write down is so dramatic that I have yet to have a patient return with a diary who wasn't simply flabbergasted by what he found himself reading after that week. Here's what a number of studies have discovered: you won't remember eating it or drinking it if you don't write it down. So write it down.

Am I repeating myself? I guess I am, but I just want to emphasize that YOU SHOULD WRITE IT ALL DOWN.

Meanwhile, I want you to keep a parallel diary of your exercise and other physical activity. As with food, we tend to avoid looking at our level of physical activity – or inactivity. Your exercise diary will give you a good overview of what level of physical activity you gravitate towards, what you enjoy and what you avoid.

STEP 2: THE PERFECT FIT QUESTIONNAIRE – TO DIET SUCCESSFULLY, KNOW THYSELF

The true secret to successful weight loss is 'Know thyself'. Know what you need, both physically and psychologically, from food and how to satisfy those needs in a way that's compatible with weight loss. Self-knowledge around our food needs is more complicated than it sounds. Perhaps nowhere do physical and emotional issues connect so deeply than in our relationship with food.

The Perfect Fit Questionnaire is an in-depth exercise in self-discovery. It is a series of 141 questions about what, when, why and how you eat. It draws upon what you know about the foods you like and the foods that make you feel full. The questionnaire systematically uncovers the obvious and not-so-obvious truths about your individual medical history, family history, and food and weight history. It investigates the exercise and stress levels in your life.

In addition to your own medical history, it asks about your parents' and siblings' medical history. There are questions about your diet and exercise history. Using that basic data, the questionnaire can identify patterns in the way you eat.

You'll see that it is broken into 20 sections of 5 to 10 questions each. Each of these sections identifies some meaningful aspect of the relationship between you and that complex calculus of intake (food) and output (activity) that describes you at your current weight. The first several sections focus on food preferences. The questions show you if you are a 'Carnimore', someone who can't imagine life without meat; a 'Dairy Queen/King', who needs the cheese with the crackers; a sweets lover; or veggie hater. All these preferences shape your current diet and will shape your perfect diet. Considering these is a key factor in determining what your diet should look like.

Then we try to figure out what makes you full. Some of my patients tell me that they can't feel full unless they eat a certain amount of food. They just aren't satisfied eating less, no matter how many calories they take in. Still others feel cravings for specific tastes or textures. They find themselves standing in front of the refrigerator scanning the shelves for . . . something. Maybe it's a food with a crunchy texture; maybe it's a taste of something sweet; maybe it's something sour or hot. If they can figure out what they are hungering for, they can eat a tiny bit of that and finally be satisfied. If not, they find themselves eating other things and, too often, still not getting that satisfied feeling. All of us have multiple ways of feeling full; figure out which ones are important for you, and you will be able to feel full and eat less by specifically directing your eating to answer that hunger.

The questionnaire also asks about your medical history. If you are healthy and under 30, then your own history may not be as important as the history of your parents or siblings. Diet and activity have a tremendous impact on your likelihood of developing many diseases that have a hereditary component to them. For example, diabetes is much more common in those with a family history of diabetes. If you are overweight or inactive, your risk is even greater. Hypertension, too, is far more common in those with a family history of high blood pressure. So medical history, both yours and your family's, will also be a factor in the diet that works best for you.

Eating habits are key in dieting. Do you skip breakfast? Do you eat only one meal a day? Do you snack? Do you need to nibble? Do you eat regular meals, or is your life too hectic to allow the traditional three square meals? Do you eat out often? Which meals? Who cooks in your household? Who shops? All of these issues will have an impact on your perfect diet.

What about emotional eating? Are you a stress eater? Do you eat when you're bored? When you're angry? When you need a reward? Understanding your eating triggers is an essential part of constructing a diet that works for you.

Finally, let's look at your level of activity. Do you always take the lift? Do you always drive to the supermarket? Are there ways to increase the amount of daily activity in your life? And what about exercise? Do you walk? Do you run? Do you swim? Have you ever exercised? Which kind? Why did you stop? What keeps you from exercising now? Being active is essential to weight loss and to weight-loss maintenance. Our job is to help you find an activity – or even better, several activities – that fits comfortably into your life.

Once you collect all this data, you're ready to score the questionnaire and find out which diet fits you best.

STEP 3: IDENTIFY WHICH BASIC DIET IS RIGHT FOR YOU

Diets that help you lose weight do so by reducing the number of calories you take in and increasing the amount of energy you use up. Having said that, different diets use different strategies to achieve those ends.

Most diets reduce your calorie intake by restricting access to one or more types of foods. Once you recognize this, it's easy to classify the vast panoply of diets onto a sort of spectrum based on what exactly they are limiting.

At one end are the very low fat (high-carbohydrate) diets such as those of Dr Dean Ornish and Dr Neal Bernard. Both recommend extraordinary reductions in fat intake. Dr Ornish recommends a vegetarian diet; Dr Bernard goes even further to recommend a vegan diet in which you eat no animal products whatsoever. A little further up the spectrum you get the more moderate fat restrictions where you're allowed to eat fat, but only the so-called good fat. These would include diets recommended by Weight Watchers, and the Eat, Drink, and Be Healthy diet as designed by Dr Walter Willett. These generally recommend that you restrict your fat intake to 30 to 35 per cent of the calories you eat.

Right smack in the middle, you get diets that focus on cutting calories. These diets come in two basic flavours. There are those that offer unlimited amounts of a few low-calorie foods. Rotation diets – like the recent cabbage soup diet – use this strategy. More commonly, calorie-counting diets focus on portion control and offer a much wider variety of foods, emphasizing foods that provide a greater sense of fullness and satisfaction with fewer calories. Usually, they promote foods that are high in fibre, low on the glycaemic load, or both. For example, Volumetrics is a calorie-counting diet, although author Barbara Rolls, PhD, talks about it in terms of calorie per volume of food or calorie density. You can eat more low-density foods than you can high-density foods.

As we move further up the spectrum, we start seeing diets that focus on limiting carbohydrates. The Zone diet, for instance, says that you should restrict your carbohydrate intake to just 40 per cent of the calories you eat in the course of a day. Protein Power is another diet that limits access to carbohydrates but wants you to replace those carbs with protein rather than fats; the South Beach Diet is very low carb in its initial stages and then recommends the gradual introduction of some fruit and whole grain foods. And finally, at the outermost edge of the spectrum, is Dr Atkins' Diet Revolution, which seeks to reduce your carb intake to the lowest you can tolerate.

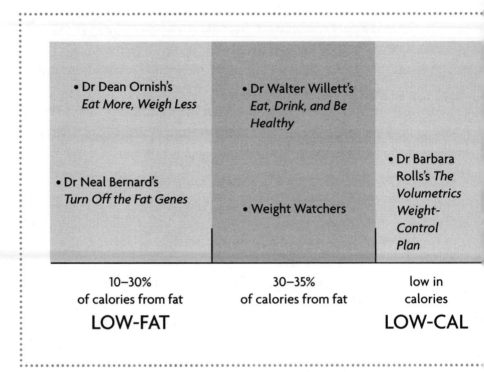

• Dr Dean Ornish's *Eat More, Weigh Less*	• Dr Walter Willett's *Eat, Drink, and Be Healthy*	• Dr Barbara Rolls's *The Volumetrics Weight-Control Plan*
• Dr Neal Bernard's *Turn Off the Fat Genes*	• Weight Watchers	
10–30% of calories from fat	30–35% of calories from fat	low in calories
LOW-FAT		**LOW-CAL**

Let's take a closer look at these many different diets. While the range might suggest that they are all arbitrary, I believe that there are particular dieters who do best on each of these diets.

So who would do well on a diet that primarily restricts fat? Let's start with food preference. Those who don't eat a lot of meat to begin with would do better than big-time Carnimores. You have to enjoy fruits and vegetables, and having a good appreciation for whole grain foods would help. Furthermore, these are people who need volume to feel full. In terms of health, I would recommend this as one possible diet for those with high cholesterol but would not recommend such a diet for those who have diabetes or who process carbohydrates abnormally. (I'll explain how to determine if you fit in this group, later, as you score the questionnaire.)

When you eat a high-carb, low-fat diet, eating regular meals is

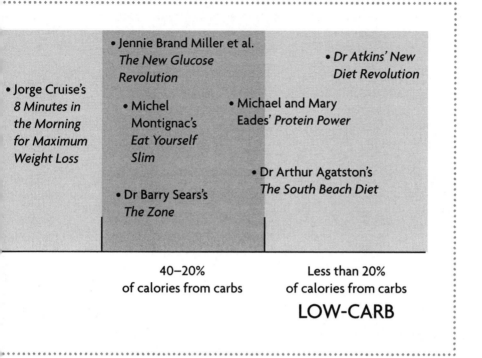

• Jennie Brand Miller et al.
*The New Glucose
Revolution*

• *Dr Atkins' New
Diet Revolution*

• Jorge Cruise's
*8 Minutes in
the Morning
for Maximum
Weight Loss*

• Michel
Montignac's
*Eat Yourself
Slim*

• Michael and Mary
Eades' *Protein Power*

• Dr Arthur Agatston's
The South Beach Diet

• Dr Barry Sears's
The Zone

40–20%
of calories from carbs

Less than 20%
of calories from carbs
LOW-CARB

particularly important since there is less fat and protein to make your feeling of fullness last. Finally, a low-fat diet is very hard to keep up with if you travel a lot and eat out frequently. Fresh fruits and veggies and whole grain foods will make up most of what you eat, and very little of that food is available away from home.

What about a calorie-counting diet? This is for people who need a lot of variety in their diets and for whom portion size is a manageable issue. If you can't eat a little of something you like, a low-calorie diet may not be for you. On the other hand, if you find yourself standing in front of the refrigerator, trying to identify the food you are craving, you may do very well on a calorie-counting diet that allows you to eat some of whatever you crave and that purposefully offers a variety of flavours and textures every day.

Finally, how about a carbohydrate-counting diet? This is a diet for eaters who enjoy meat, cheese and eggs and find it hard to feel full without them. It helps if you don't care much about variety; because you often end up eating very much the same food every day. You have to be able to live in a world with limited fruits and vegetables. And of course you have to say goodbye to breads, pastas and desserts. It is a very restrictive diet, and yet there are many who have successfully lost weight on this diet and can maintain their weight using these principles. Portion control is an important aspect of this diet, too, although it may be less of an issue because of the filling quality of proteins and fats. People who travel or eat out a lot often do well on this type of diet, because easily available main courses of grilled meat, chicken or fish plus a salad make up the pro-totypical meal of this diet.

After you figure out which sort of diet is right for you, I'll instruct you to turn to the section about that diet in part 3. There, I give a brief summary of the principles of each diet. After that is a list of foods that work with that diet and a 7-day eating plan to help you implement the diet in your own home. I have developed a version of each diet based on my own research. In general, the meal plans I recommend are rich in fresh fruits and vegetables and feature foods that are low in saturated fats and that have a low glycaemic load. Following the diet and food recommendations in your Perfect Fit Diet plan, you will have the fundamentals of the low-fat, low-calorie, or low-carbohy-drate diet that will work for you.

STEP 4: CUSTOMIZE YOUR BASIC DIET TO YOUR FOOD PREFERENCES AND MEDICAL HISTORY

Once you figure out which diet is best for you, you can shape it even further based on how you answer the individual sections of the questionnaire. Each section is designed to help you define a specific aspect of the way you eat. Once you have defined the various aspects of your diet, I will try to help you tailor your diet around this aspect that is uniquely you.

Food preferences. Food preference plays a role in customizing your diet. All classes of foods have some good in them. Our job is to look at the kinds of foods you like and understand what's good in these foods and what's not so good. Using that knowledge, you can customize your diet to maximize the healthy qualities of the foods you love while minimizing those qualities that are less healthy.

In a diet that tries, as this one does, to outsmart the forces that help us put on weight and make it hard to lose it, there can be no forbidden foods. All is allowed, but you have to plan for it. I think what too many people do is simply decide to say no to a food that they love but believe has contributed to their inability to control their weight. They decide that this food – say, a treat that is sweet or salty, filled with sugar or fat or both – may never be eaten again.

Two things happen when you do that: first, when you eat the thing that you love, it will be unplanned – you won't have any room left in your diet for it. And that's what usually happens. When you forbid yourself from having something, you end up eating it on top of everything else you eat. That doesn't work. Since you are going to have it, you need to count it, and the only real way to do that is to plan for it.

Something else happens when you know that a food is off-limits: that knowledge often drives you to eat too much of it, since you feel that you will never be able to eat it again. This is one of the ways that dieting changes your relationship to food, and one that can be avoided. If you are going to incorporate a new way of eating into your life, which I hope is your goal, you have to figure out some way to make peace with the foods you love and feel you shouldn't eat. This is one of the goals of customizing your diet.

Medical history. Your medical and family history must play a role in customizing your diet. For example, if you have a family history of high cholesterol, chances are you will not end up on a carbohydrate-counting diet based on your initial diet selection. In addition, there are ways to shape your diet so that the fats you eat will help you bring down rather than ratchet up your cholesterol.

STEP 5: CUSTOMIZE YOUR BASIC DIET TO FIT YOUR LIFESTYLE

What you eat, how you eat and when you eat are all part of your lifestyle. And despite what we nutrition buffs would like to think, chances are, they are not the most important issues of your life, but must compete with other compelling aspects of your day: your job, your family and all the other pleasures and obligations that make up a life. But the life into which you integrate this diet will have a profound effect on how it works. Therefore, you need to take your real life into consideration when you design your diet.

Usually, when a diet gets out of hand and causes weight gain, it is due not only to the foods eaten but also to when, where, why and how the food is eaten. As adults, overcommitted, wildly busy, terrifically stressed, we have developed eating habits that interfere with natural mechanisms that regulate when and how much we eat. Normally, we eat a variety of foods but take in more or less the same number of calories per day. We haven't figured out the mechanism yet – there are probably many different and overlapping ones. But thanks to this very finely tuned system, we are usually able to regulate our intake without even thinking about it so that it doesn't vary more than 100 calories or so day in and day out.

But many of the ways we eat undermine these mechanisms. Stressed-out and busy workers or parents can find themselves too busy to eat. Maybe they grab a quick snack, or maybe they just ignore the hunger pangs, but in either case chances are that when their next meal rolls around, they are starving. They sit down and in an instant consume their entire meal and more – often much more. The mechanisms that might otherwise tell them they have had enough are silenced by their outsized hunger, and they overeat. Sound familiar?

And then there is the opposite problem: some people eat when they aren't hungry. Maybe they are stressed, bored or tired – but they are not hungry. The body treats these snacks differently from the snacks you eat when you are hungry. Snacks you eat when you are hungry usually cause you to eat less at your next meal than you otherwise would eat. Snacks that you eat when you are not hungry don't do that. Your body just doesn't count them when it's doing the maths about how many calories you've eaten. So food you eat when you're not hungry ends up being just extra calories.

If you travel frequently, your food choices are limited by what is available to travellers – and those are often some sad choices. Your diet has to make room for your travel. Even if you are not on the road a lot, you may eat out frequently. Again, this is a challenge when you are trying to control what you eat. Your diet has to make room for eating out – it's as simple as that.

Working long hours often leaves us feeling that there is no time to take care of ourselves. While we can't add to the 24 hours that make up our day, in every life there has to be room to eat and drink and exercise, and while choices may be limited, there are still choices. This book will help you know which choices will work best for you.

I also hope I'm able to persuade you that one of those choices will be to integrate a higher level of activity into your life. You can lose weight without exercising. Many studies support that. But it's much harder to *maintain* weight loss without exercise, and many studies support that as well. I know that exercise can seem silly and too difficult to integrate into a busy life, but there is every reason in the world to believe that it is a necessary part of a healthy life, so it needs to be part of yours. Our job is to figure out a way for you to sneak some exercise into your leisure. To do this, find the activities that suit you and emphasize those. I can't promise you that exercise will help you lose weight, but I can promise that it will make you feel better and that *that* will help you lose weight.

HOW THE PERFECT FIT DIET WORKS: SHELLEY

So, how does this work in real life? Let's go back to my sister Shelley. She's 48 years old and has been overweight for most of her life. When she found out that I was putting this questionnaire together, she begged me to let her be the first person to try it.

So, I assigned her homework – create a food diary and collect her basic medical info – and then we reconnoitred.

Steps 1 and 2: The Eating Diary and the Questionnaire

As we went through her food diary, once again I was reminded of how useful and instructive this exercise is. I say this even though I know my sister very well.

Except for a couple of years just before puberty, we have always been the best of friends. Even though we haven't lived near each other since school, we talk almost daily and visit frequently. I bet I know her better than anyone else on earth. And I'd say she knows me just as well. But I got a whole new education about my sister by going through this diary.

Over the years, when we've spoken about diets, she has always raved about the low-carb Scarsdale diet or the Atkins diet. Because of that, I just assumed that she ate a lot of meat and not so many veggies. Wrong.

She did eat meat every day, often at two meals, but she also ate lots of carbs – fruits, pasta, salads. Going on a low-carb diet, which had worked in the past, was going to be a big change for her. And a big change means probably not sustainable – her history supported this.

When I asked her about these low-carb diets she's had success with in the past, she made an astonishing admission – at least astonishing to me. She admitted that one of the reasons that low-carb diets worked for her was because they were so very different from her usual pattern of eating. That difference somehow helped her remember that she was supposed to be losing weight. Also, they prohibited some of the things that she had a hard time modulating, like sweets. And – something else I didn't know about my sister – she thought it was easier to give up sweets than to learn to moderate them. So these diets, by prohibiting all carbs, allowed her to avoid the sweets she so often craved – at least for a while.

But, not surprisingly, sweets did show up in her food diary. She had a clear weakness for cookies, chocolate and something called a McFlurry.

Another important clue to which diet she should go on: when asked what she most valued in her diet, she said food variety – it was more important than eating more food and more important than eating rich foods.

Step 3: Identify Which Basic Diet Plan Is the Right One

When you add all that together – lots of meat at meal times, lots of carbs, a passion for sweets and a need for variety – it becomes clear what kind of diet would suit Shelley best: a diet that counts calories. One that allows her to eat all kinds of foods, just not too much. A 1,200-calorie diet would allow her to lose 450–900g (1–2lb) per week, and when she approached her target weight, she could increase that slowly to a 1,500-calorie diet to maintain her weight.

Step 4: Customize the Basic Diet to Food Preferences and Medical History

Food preference was pretty clear: Shelley was a Carnimore, someone who likes to eat meat daily; she was also a 'Vegecarian', big into fresh fruits and vegetables. She loved pasta, so she was a 'Starch Stealer'. Finally, she was a 'Sweets Eater' and needed to make room in her diet for an occasional taste of something sweet. We talked about how to incorporate each of these foods into her diet. She liked variety and was sure to get lots of it; the biggest concern for her was going to be portion control.

You also need to customize for medical history. For Shelley, this was pretty easy. Her Body Mass Index (BMI) was 28, which isn't too bad (25–29 is overweight; 30 plus is obese) and her waist was 76cm (30in). (Women with waists greater than 89cm/35in are at increased risk of heart disease.) She had no chronic diseases: her blood pressure ran in the 100/70 range, and her cholesterol was well controlled with a low LDL and high HDL. She's never had any surgery, and she took no medications. She didn't drink or smoke. She lives with her husband and her dog.

Her family history was also good. There's no history of heart disease, high blood pressure or diabetes in anyone. These are important questions, since if you have any of these illnesses or risk factors, you have to recognize that you're at increased risk of heart disease. She doesn't, so at least until menopause, these aren't important issues in her diet.

Step 5: Customize the Basic Diet to Fit the Lifestyle

My sister runs a small but growing business out of her own home, and she has maybe five full-time employees and anywhere from five to ten part-timers. Like all small-business owners, she finds running her own business exciting and stressful.

Most weekdays, she doesn't have breakfast – just a cup of coffee with skimmed milk. She doesn't snack; so by the time lunch rolls around, she's pretty hungry. Her kitchen is right next to the office, which could be convenient, but she doesn't like to cook when her employees are there, and she feels self-conscious about eating in front of them too. So most days she goes out for lunch with her husband, who also runs his own business from home.

She doesn't have an afternoon snack and often works late after her employees have gone home. She and her husband usually eat late and eat out for dinner – maybe four nights a week.

Snacks are often grabbed on the way out the door or in the car when a meal has been missed. Stress eating usually occurs in the early evening as she's winding up the business of the day and is alone in the office.

Exercise helps with the stress, but when the stress is highest, she complains, she has the least time to exercise. When she does exercise, she either catches an aerobics class at a nearby gym or jogs on a treadmill at home. She likes to exercise at lunchtime but often doesn't have time for it.

Based on Shelley's answers about her lifestyle, the Perfect Fit Questionnaire recommended the following:

1. Eat three meals a day with healthy snacks available for between-meal hunger.
2. Try not to ignore your hunger until you are famished. Eat when you are hungry, not when you are starving.

3. While you are working to lose weight, limit your eating out to one or two meals per week.

4. When you do go out to eat, order a juice or light soup as an appetizer, then order only a small appetizer for the main course. If that won't be enough, order a small salad as well.

5. On the weekends, prepare food ahead that will be easy to warm up on those tired evenings when you just can't cook.

6. Keep track of what you eat every day; tally the calories at the end of each meal. Continue the food diary.

7. Prepare your menu for the week on Sunday and prepare as much of it as you can ahead of time.

8. Have a target number of calories for 2 or 3 days – not just per day – so that you can accommodate good days and bad days.

9. Build variety into your exercise plan. Find an aerobics class that fits your schedule and use that at least 2 or 3 days per week.

10. Exercise at home (on your treadmill) on days when you're too busy to go out to exercise.

So that's how it should work with my sister. So far, so good. After the first 6 weeks, she lost 4.5kg (10lb) and was feeling pretty good. She started closing her business for a half an hour each day for lunch so she can eat with her staff or exercise, and that's been good for everyone. But, as we all know, it's not how well you start the diet but how well you can stick with the diet. That, only time will tell. But since her diet is now customized to satisfy her personal food cravings, she's likely to succeed for the long term.

HOW THE PERFECT FIT DIET WORKS: MATT

Matt is a 40-year-old businessman with short, cropped dark curls and deep dimples. Although he'd been an athlete at university, marriage and a successful career had cut the time he was able to work out, and he had piled the weight on. As of a year ago, he weighed 128kg (20 stone), and his cholesterol was high. But then his father died suddenly of a massive heart attack, and Matt realized that he could be next if he didn't lose weight. Over the course of the next year, Matt lost almost 45kg (7 stone) by working out every day and obsessively limiting his calories to 800 calories a day. When he got within 9kg (20lb) of his dream weight of 72.5kg (11½ stone), he was elated.

But almost immediately, he began to put the weight back on. When he passed 90kg (14 stone), he became frantic, desperate. Every day he would pledge to limit his calories to less than 800 a day; most days he ate three or four times that many. He couldn't bring himself to work out, because he hated to see how he looked in shorts. He even tried to make himself vomit after a binge when he ate the icing off a huge rectangular cake, then threw out the rest of the cake. That's when he knew he needed help. His question was, 'How can I stop this yo-yoing and maintain a reasonable weight?'

Steps 1 and 2: The Eating Diary and Questionnaire

Matt weighed 90kg (14 stone) at 1.72m (5ft 8in), which gave him a BMI of 30. He already exercised pretty regularly, lifting weights 3 days a week. He ate a good breakfast of fruit and porridge every morning. Lunch at the office was a small salad, dried beans, or dried soup, and he fixed a pretty healthy dinner most nights of the week for himself, his wife and his two teenage daughters.

What he ate at mealtime was low-fat and high-carbohydrate and in small portions. He usually had chicken or fish. Lots of potatoes. Huge amounts of fruit. Good fibre content. So why was he overweight? It was what he ate between mealtimes. As a big-time executive, he found himself going out to lunch three times per week. But beyond that, Matt was a stress eater. Matt's preference was chocolate, and there was plenty of it in his office. When the stress was on, Matt would wander through the office, talking with various people about whatever the problem was and all the time munching chocolate that he seemed to find just about everywhere.

At home, Matt had a different problem: after dinner, Matt often found himself sitting in front of the TV eating biscuits, crackers, nuts, whatever he could find.

In terms of health, Matt was doing pretty well. He had high cholesterol but his blood pressure was good. He didn't smoke, drank only occasionally and exercised regularly. His mum was still alive and in great shape.

Step 3: Identify Which Basic Diet Plan Is the Right One

Based on what Matt already ate, and since he was a middle-age man with high cholesterol and fat which accumulated around his waist (the most dangerous kind of fat), I knew he would do well with a low-fat diet. The questionnaire showed the same. For that he needed to restrict his fat intake to 30 to 33 per cent of his calories with less than 7 per cent coming from saturated fats. The only oil he should use is olive oil or other monounsaturated oils like rapeseed, or polyunsaturated oil like corn oil.

Step 4: Customize the Basic Diet to Food Preferences and Medical History

Matt eats lots of potatoes but avoids the leafy greens we usually recommend. Most likely he's a PROP taster (more on that later) and is avoiding vegetables with even a trace of bitterness in them. I directed him to vegetables that he hadn't listed in his food diary but that he might enjoy if he were a PROP taster. I told him to eat more artichokes, asparagus, avocado, carrots, sweetcorn, squash and eat more fruits, which he seems to love. He also loves rice and beans, which is very helpful on a low-fat diet. I asked him to consider rice and bean dishes as a main course at least two times per week. Experiment with soya products like tofu. Use whole-grain pastas.

Step 5: Customize the Basic Diet to Fit the Lifestyle

Matt eats out a lot and feels compelled to clean his plate – training that starts early and is hard to get over. My advice to him is the same as my advice to Shelley: when you are trying to lose weight, limit eating out to one or two meals per week. And when you do eat out, order a light soup or juice, and then an appetizer or even two. Avoid bread. Avoid alcohol.

More importantly: Matt lets himself get too hungry between breakfast and supper. It is particularly important on a low-fat diet to eat three meals a day and have healthy snacks available. Don't ignore your hunger until you are starving. Eat when you are hungry.

On days he doesn't go out to lunch, Matt starves himself with small meals. He's proud of the fact that most days he eats less than 500 calories (in meals) before getting home from work. Clearly, he needs more that that. No wonder he runs around his office munching on everyone's chocolate – he's starving. He needs to eat three real meals a day and planned snacks as needed. That way other people's snacks won't be so tempting.

Matt clearly needs a bigger lunch. He also needs one that combines foods. He's eating all carbohydrates for his lunch and clearly that's not satisfying him. He needs a lunch that combines carbs with more filling proteins and, if he has a sweet tooth, something wholesome like a piece of fruit. And if he gets hungry after lunch, he should eat an afternoon snack before he goes home and starts cooking.

Finally, he needs to stop that late-night noshing in front of the TV. Matt is not alone – eating and watching TV seems to have become a very popular pastime. But unfortunately the combination of inactivity and increased calorie intake is compounded by the fact that the majority of foods TV ads encourage us to eat are foods that are of low nutritional value – better known as junk foods. (In the UK a survey into food commercials aimed at youngsters found that 99 per cent of the food and drink advertised had either a high fat, high sugar or high salt content.) With this type of constant reminder, no wonder those activities get linked together. Plus if Matt eats more food earlier in the day, the need to nosh will diminish. But the habit of watching and eating will remain unless he forces himself out of it.

On the other hand, Matt's exercise level is pretty good. He lifts weights three times a week. Hard to improve on that. But I recommended that he add another exercise to his repertoire – maybe cycling or running on the days he doesn't lift – to give him more of an aerobic workout. Those who like to exercise should build a variety of exercises into their schedule.

Matt made great progress from the start. On a 33-per-cent-fat diet and his fabulous exercise habit, he lost about 6.8kg (15lb) over 4 months. He's happy there, and his weight has remained stable.

So how's he doing it? Lunch is working well. He reports that he has a kitchen at his office and once a week or so he shops for stuff to keep in the kitchen for lunch. He uses the time he spends making lunch to think stuff over. His biggest crisis came a couple of months ago when he changed jobs. With the new job came new obligations to lunch out and, of course, new stress. He's found a restaurant in the area that serves low-fat food that he likes. And he's found a couple of appetizers that work as a meal for him.

He's also enjoyed the variety in his exercise plan. He now swims a couple of times a week and cycles with his kids at the weekends.

And he's healthier too. His cholesterol is down so much that his doctor took him off his medicine. He feels more energetic, happier, sexier. And since he's the household cook, his wife has lost 6.8kg (15lb) and she's feeling good too.

WHAT THE PERFECT FIT DIET CAN DO FOR YOU

Shelley and Matt are typical of the formerly failed dieters I meet every week in my clinical practice. They see their lapses as proof of their weak wills. But dieting isn't about moral strength – its about compatibility between diet and dieter. Finding the diet that fits you requires that marriage I keep talking about between what science can teach us about dieting and what we know about ourselves. My five-step strategy will lead you to the diet that is right for you.

My patients have done it. You can too.

PART

THE PERFECT FIT QUESTIONNAIRE

BEFORE YOU GET STARTED on the questionnaire, you will have to do a little research. You know you will need to keep a food and exercise diary. You will also have to gather other types of data about yourself and your family. You will probably have to contact your doctor to answer some of the questions I ask about your health.

Specifically, you will need to know:

- Your blood pressure
- Your levels of total cholesterol, LDL cholesterol, HDL cholesterol and triglycerides (these are measured as part of the standard cholesterol test, otherwise known as the standard lipid panel)
- Your fasting blood sugar
- What medicines you take and what they are for

Your doctor will probably be perfectly happy to take your blood pressure and do a cholesterol test but you may need to pay to have your blood sugar levels tested. If you are over the age of 30 or if you are younger than 30 but have high blood pressure, diabetes, or are a smoker, you should develop your Perfect Fit Diet from this book, but consult with your doctor before you begin.

You also need to know about the medical problems of your immediate family. Does your mother, father, sister or brother have high blood pressure, diabetes or high cholesterol? These chronic diseases tend to run in families, and if your parents have them, then you are at a higher risk of getting them too. Does anyone in your immediate family have heart disease such as angina or coronary artery disease, or have any of them had a heart attack? Heart disease runs in families as well, and children of a parent who had a heart attack at a young age (under 45 for a man and under 55 for a woman) are at increased risk themselves of heart disease.

One last piece of information you will need to know about yourself is your waist size. Women who have a waist that is 88cm (35in) or greater, and men who have a waist size of 102cm (40in) or greater are at increased risk of heart disease and diabetes and may have a condition known as metabolic syndrome. This group of symptoms suggests that the way you metabolize carbohydrates is abnormal, and this has a definite impact on the type of diet that would be best for you. When you have all this information available, you will be ready to fill in the questionnaire.

One last word: when you fill out this questionnaire, try to be as honest as possible. The temptation is to lie to yourself – but be honest. This is where it matters. As I've said from the beginning, the Perfect Fit Diet combines what science knows about weight loss with what you know about yourself. Over the doorway to the Oracle of Delphi, there were carved only two words: Know Thyself. That is where all truth, redemption and revelation begin.

4 CHAPTER

YOUR EATING AND EXERCISE DIARY

◆

'Knowledge is power.'

— FRANCIS BACON

SO FAR, I'VE JUST BEEN TALKING about the theories behind this book – what I have learned from my research about diets and appetites and dieters like you. A quick summary:

1. All diets do work – for some people.

2. An individual's optimal diet, your diet, will be determined by many factors: genetic, environmental, personal.

3. The science of satiety – what satisfies you – is still a young field, but it's beginning to reveal that much of what we need to satisfy us is hardwired.

4. Diet and lifestyle are not easily changed and even when they are, that change is difficult to maintain.

5. Getting out of shape did not happen overnight. Getting back into shape won't either.

6. The best diet for you will be the one that comes closest to fitting you as you are.

That's the theory. Now we need to move on to that second part – what you know about yourself.

Take my analogy of diet and lifestyle being like a piece of clothing. You can buy it off the shelf – we often do. But if it's important that the dress or jacket fit perfectly, we often have to tailor it to make it fit just right. The most important tool a tailor has is his tape measure. That tells him what he needs to know about your body and how to make the garment fit. Your eating and exercise diary will be your tape measure in tailoring your diet.

You know what your body looks like, in general. Maybe you know that you have broad shoulders or long legs, but do you know exactly how broad, how long? Probably not. Same with your diet. You have an idea about what you eat and why you eat it. You have a feeling about how active you are, but you can't really quantify it. Your eating and exercise diary will let you measure what you think you know – but don't know well enough to help you find the diet that is perfect for you.

You can't make a suit without knowing your measurements. You can't pick a diet without knowing what you eat.

Of course, you probably think you know what you eat. Be prepared to surprise yourself. There have been lots of studies that show that food recall – that is, just asking people what they eat – is a very poor way to discover the truth about diet. It's not just that people lie, although that may be part of it. It's that most people just don't remember everything they put in their mouths.

Let's look at what the research shows. In a study done a few years ago, researchers had 36 women spend a single day and night in a special hospital ward. Everything they ate was secretly recorded. At the end of the 24-hour period, the women were asked to write down everything they ate while they were there.

They couldn't do it.

They thought they could do it, but when their lists were compared with the lists of what they actually ate, it was clear that the women weren't nearly as accurate as they thought they were. They could remember some of what they ate at mealtime, but not everything, and they were terrible at remembering how much they ate. Even more notably, virtually all the women frequently forgot what they ate that *wasn't* part of a meal. No one could remember their snacks.

That's why you need a diary.

When my sister Shelley decided to start this diet, I gave her the whole rap about how she needed to write down everything she ate in order for us to figure out how she should eat to lose weight. She was totally on board, ready, even excited.

When she brought back her diary and her questionnaire, she had a confession to make: she had originally filled out the questionnaire without keeping the diary. She considered herself a reasonable person, someone capable of honestly remembering and reporting what she ate. And she thought that keeping the diary was just too tough and too time consuming. She was anxious to start the diet.

So she filled out the questionnaire as best she could. And she *is* a reasonable person. This is how reasonable she is: when she looked the questionnaire over, she realized that what she wrote down couldn't possibly represent everything she'd eaten within the past week because if it did, she'd have just about starved to death.

'I knew that I had left things off my list,' she confessed to me later, 'but I couldn't remember or even imagine what they were.'

So she started to keep the diary. It was a little tough – especially when she had to write down things she felt she 'shouldn't have eaten'. But she did it.

When she sat down to fill out the questionnaire again, she got an education. She saw what she had left out when she had tried to fill it out without an eating diary. She was surprised, but also interested. 'It wasn't just the bad stuff I left off the list, although that was a lot of it.' She noticed two types of foods she omitted. The first was foods she didn't think she ate – her example: baked goods. 'When I got to that part of the questionnaire the first time, it was a no-brainer. I never eat baked goods – cakes, cookies. Not what I like. But when I kept my diary, I saw that I did eat quite a few baked goods – muffins and even a couple of cookies. I couldn't believe it, but there it was in black and white.'

Another error she noticed when she compared her first questionnaire with her second was that she, like the people in the study, was pretty good at remembering what she ate at meals, but snacks just fell off her radar. 'If you had asked me if I ate snacks, I would have said that I didn't normally. Actually keeping this diary made me realize that in one day – and this actually happened twice during the week I kept my diary – I ate as much in snacks as I did meals. It blew my mind.'

'When I looked at the second questionnaire, it was a little embarrassing, but I knew it was a better picture of my diet than the first one. The first one was what I thought I ate, and really what I wished I ate. The second one was what I *really* ate.'

Keeping a diary isn't just the best reality check for people like Shelley. Scientific research confirms that it's the most reliable method of tracking what we eat. In one UK study, more than 100 men and women were asked to write down everything they ate for 1 week. Actually, they were asked to do it twice – the second time 1 year after the first time – in part because the researchers wanted to see how much their diets changed.

Since the participants weren't living in a hospital for all this time, the researchers needed some other way of checking out the accuracy of their eating diaries. So, using the principle that what goes in must come out, they asked the participants to keep all of their urine for one entire day – they did this several times over the course of a year – and the scientists analySed it for some of the essential components of the diet that would be excreted in the urine. They then compared the foods listed in the diaries with those that showed up in the urine. They found that diaries were pretty good at recording what was eaten. Not 100 per cent, but not bad. And much better than asking people what they ate and relying on their selective memory.

HOW TO KEEP AN EATING AND EXERCISE DIARY

First, I want you to keep your diary for a week. Why 7 days? Because that's probably how long it takes to get a flavour for the variation in your diet over the workweek and weekend. There's also a phenomenon in which just the act of keeping a diary changes the way some people eat. It's Heisenberg's uncertainty principle applied to food. Heisenberg proved that looking at an object – his objects were very tiny – changed that object. Well, the same kind of thing happens on a more human scale when you try to capture what you eat. Just knowing that you'll have to write it down changes your eating habits, at least for a while. In order to record what you usually eat, you have to keep a diary long enough to catch yourself eating normally.

Let's go back to the 100 men and women mentioned opposite who kept diaries. Researchers found that their subjects had done a pretty good job of writing down what they ate – but the scientists realized that their subjects had to be eating more food than they listed. How did they know? The same way Shelley knew: because if they had eaten only the foods that they listed, then they wouldn't weigh what they weighed. So, they figured that their subjects underestimated how much they ate. And this has been noted in other studies – that because people don't usually report enough calories consumed to maintain their present weight, researchers believe that these people tend to underestimate how much they eat. Even more damning – overweight people tend to underestimate more than normal-weight people.

For many years, researchers extrapolated from this that everyone lies about what they eat. But a cleverly designed study revealed a different phenomenon. In a study conducted in the Netherlands, researchers asked 30 overweight men to write down everything they ate for the week. They also measured weight and metabolic rate several times over the course of a week. Here's what they found: the men were writing down just about everything they ate. But they were eating less than they normally did. And they lost weight. Just the act of keeping a diary made these men – and presumably just about everyone who keeps a diet diary – eat less. This change in eating habits accounted for an estimated 70 per cent of the 'underreporting'. An earlier study done with thin women showed the same thing: their apparent underreporting came from their eating less when they were keeping a diary. And the shorter the time period covered by the diary, the more extreme the underreporting.

Keeping the diary for a week allows for much of this. After a few days of self-conscious eating, you'll revert to your true eating habits. That's what we need to capture. Which is why *keeping a week-long record is your first principle as food diarist*.

The second is: *when you write down what you ate, write down what time you ate it as well*. If you aren't a watch-wearing person, estimate the time. Just the hour is fine. This way you will see when you get hungry, or at least when you eat.

Third, *write down what you ate right then, right as you are eating it*. Don't wait until the end of the day to summarize what you ate, because then you are trusting your memory, and I hope I have convinced you that your memory can't be trusted for information like this. You need to keep your diary with you at all times, because you never know when you are going to eat or drink something, and you need to write it down as soon as you consume it.

Fourth, *I want you to write down how much you ate as soon as you've eaten it*. I don't expect you to weigh or measure everything you eat, but I want you to estimate the amount. Did you have a handful of crisps or the whole bag? Was it a single-serving bag or the economy-size giant bag? Did you have half a biscuit or 10 biscuits? You're the only person who's ever going to read this diary, so you might as well give yourself the benefit of accurate information about what you eat.

Finally, and this is hard, but also very important, *I want you to write down why you ate*. Sure, sometimes we eat because we are hungry. Often, however, there is a different reason. Find out what those reasons are. You might be surprised at what you'll discover about yourself. Some people eat when they are worried or angry. Others eat when they are happy. Some people eat when they see something they like. Other people eat because they are bored. Sometimes people eat out of habit. Often people eat when they are stressed, when they are fidgety, when they are wildly busy. Some people eat when they need comfort.

There are probably as many reasons to eat when you are not hungry as there are people, so find out what makes you eat. It will help you lose the weight you want to lose, and keep it off.

Turn to page 64 to see what a completed eating diary page might look like.

You will also need to document your exercise and activity level. Exercise, you know what that is. Just write down what you do, how long you did it, and whether or not you became out of breath while doing it. The activity part isn't so intuitive. Activity is really anything you do that requires you to move in a sustained manner. Going to the bathroom from the living room – not really an activity. Walking up two flights of stairs at work, that is activity. Housework, gardening, walking to the station or across a large car park – those would all count as activities. Write them down as often as you can so that you can see how active you are on a daily basis. I also want you to rate your exertion. If you walked across a car park and didn't get out of breath, that's a 1. If you walked up a flight or two of steps and you didn't break into a sweat, but you were breathing a little hard, that's a 2. And if you ran to catch your bus, but the driver didn't see you right away so you actually broke out in a sweat, give yourself a 3. See page 67 for an example of how an exercise diary should look.

Just a couple of words before I send you off on this task. Keeping a diary is hard work. I can't tell you exactly why, but it is. Part of it, sure, is just doing something you don't normally do

(continued on page 66)

＊

DAY 1: Day of Week   Monday

(Rate your hunger on a scale of 0 to 3: 0 = not hungry; 3 = very hungry.)

MORNING

Time   6:30

What You Ate or Drank   coffee with milk and sugar

Where You Ate or Drank   in my kitchen

Why You Ate or Drank/Hunger Level   Habit – 0

Time   7:15

What You Ate or Drank   muffin, bought from the petrol station

Where You Ate or Drank   in the car on the way to work

Why You Ate or Drank/Hunger Level   needed a snack – 1

Time   9:15

What You Ate or Drank   biscuits from the office biscuit tin, coffee with milk and sugar

Where You Ate or Drank   office

Why You Ate or Drank/Hunger Level   free food! – 0

MIDDAY

Time   1:30

What You Ate or Drank   chicken Caesar salad, 2 white rolls, diet coke, coffee with milk

Where You Ate or Drank   TGIF

Why You Ate or Drank/Hunger Level   HUNGRY! – 3

Time   2:30

What You Ate or Drank   chocolates

Where You Ate or Drank   office

Why You Ate or Drank/Hunger Level   they were there! – 0

EVENING

Time   6:30

What You Ate or Drank   beer and honey-roasted peanuts, approx. 1 handful

Where You Ate or Drank   pub

Why You Ate or Drank/Hunger Level   needed a drink after 3-hour meeting in office – 1

Time   7:15

What You Ate or Drank   pasta primavera with Parmesan cheese, diet coke, red wine (2 glasses), garlic bread

Where You Ate or Drank   home

Why You Ate or Drank/Hunger Level   Decided to eat with the kids early, even though I wasn't really hungry – 1

in the midst of your very busy day. It's not easy to integrate new practices into your routine. But I suspect it's more than that.

There is something about eating, especially if you weigh more than you want to weigh, something very emotional. And this emotional component makes us reluctant to even know about what we eat, much less write it down. I know that even though I don't have a problem with my weight, I have difficulty writing down what I eat. My patients – the ones who are honest, in any case – also acknowledge that it is tough, really tough.

But – and this is important too – keeping a diary will give you information you didn't have before, information that you can use to change your diet and lifestyle in a way that will fit you perfectly.

Losing weight is not just a matter of eating less, but keeping it off – that's the trick. Making the transformation from periodic dieter to someone who has a diet that does what she wants it to do takes more than just any diet. It takes the diet that's best for you, and the only way to come up with that is to understand your body and your feelings about what you eat and why.

This diary is the key to learning about what you like and what you think and feel about the foods you eat. Change without direction or understanding – which is all that any off-the-shelf diet has to offer – is change that's going to be hard to maintain. That's why this job of keeping a diary will be the hardest job you'll ever come to love.

ACTIVITY AND EXERCISE DIARY

✳

Rate your exertion on a scale of 1 to 3.
1 = no sweat, breathing easily
2 = no sweat, breathing hard
3 = sweat dripping, out of breath

MORNING

Time   8:30

Activity or Exercise   had trouble parking, so ended up walking a couple of streets to work

Duration and Level of Exertion   5 minutes, level 1

Time   9:00

Activity or Exercise   lift slow, so walked down 2 flights of stairs. Walked back up after mtg

Duration and Level of Exertion   2 minutes, level 1 . . . 3 minutes, level 2

Time   11:30

Activity or Exercise   walked to restaurant, was late, so walked pretty fast

Duration and Level of Exertion   10 minutes, level 2

5 CHAPTER

YOUR PERFECT
FIT QUESTIONNAIRE

THE HEART OF THE PERFECT FIT DIET is this questionnaire. I'm going to ask you questions about what you eat, how you eat it and how you feel about it. I'm going to ask you about how you have dieted in the past: what worked, what didn't, what you craved, why you stopped. I'm going to ask you about your parents' health and yours too. And I'm going to ask you about the activity in your life.

There are a lot of questions simply because how we eat, how we exercise and how our bodies react are complicated and shaped by many forces. This test will help you figure out your Perfect Fit Diet by trying to take as many of those complex factors into consideration as possible.

Let's do a quick inventory of what you will need to complete this questionnaire. Check these off as you collect the information.

- You have your food diary that reports everything you have eaten or drunk for a total of 7 days and your 7-day activity diary.
- You've got your blood pressure, fasting glucose and cholesterol profile.
- You've called your parents or siblings to find out what types of chronic illness your parents had.
- You have a tape measure to determine your waist size.

As you fill out the questionnaire, you will notice that it's broken up into sections. Each set of questions has been developed to evaluate specific aspects of your diet and your preferences. You're going to have to keep track of your answers, so I have left spaces for you to fill in your answer. You will need to total your score at the end of each section. If you can't bring yourself to write in a book, get a piece of lined paper and number it from 1 to 141 and record your answers there. Or better yet, photocopy the model answer sheet I have included just after the questionnaire.

At the end of each section, there is a little grading system for it. Most sections will give you two types of answers: one will be part of a cumulative score that directs you to one of the three main diet plans. At the very end of each section you will see a line where you can mark which diet that part of the questionnaire recommends for you. You will give yourself a point in either the Counting Carbohydrates column (CCarbs), the Counting Calories (CCals) column, or the Counting Fats column (CFats). When you finish, you will tally up your points for each diet, and the one that gets the most will be the one most likely to suit you perfectly.

The other type of answer will be a score that will help you customize your diet based on specific aspects of your food preferences, family and medical history, and dieting history. You can do the sections one at a time and score yourself at the end of each, or you can plough through to the end and then calculate your two scores.

THE QUESTIONNAIRE

Please answer the following questions. Some will ask you to look at your food diary; others will be based on what you know about yourself. Keep in mind that there are no right or wrong answers; only *your* answers. This isn't about whether the way you eat is healthy; this test is about how you eat, period.

◆

'From principles is derived probability,
but truth or certainty is obtained only from facts.'
— NATHANIEL HAWTHORNE

◆

'Just the facts, ma'am.'
— JOE FRIDAY, *DRAGNET*

FOOD PREFERENCES

Please answer these questions based on your 7-day diary.

Meat and Eggs

1. How often did you eat chicken over the past week?

    a. Never

    b. 1 to 3 times

    c. 4 to 6 times

    d. Daily

                                                                1._____

2. How often did you eat beef or veal over the past week?

    a. Never

    b. 1 to 3 times

    c. 4 to 6 times

    d. Daily

2. _____

3. How often did you eat fish or seafood over the past week?

    a. Never

    b. 1 to 3 times

    c. 4 to 6 times

    d. Daily

3. _____

4. How often did you eat pork over the past week?

    a. Never

    b. 1 to 3 times

    c. 4 to 6 times

    d. Daily

4. _____

5. How often did you eat any other meat or poultry over the past week?

    a. Never

    b. 1 to 3 times

    c. 4 to 6 times

    d. Daily

5. _____

6. How often did you eat eggs over the past week?

    a. Never

    b. 1 to 3 times

c. 4 to 6 times

d. Daily

6. _____

Scoring 1 to 6: Give yourself 1 point for every *a*, 5 for every *b*, 10 for every *c*, and 20 for every *d*.

Total: _____

If you have a score greater than 20, then perhaps you are a Carnimore. For details on how to work with your basic carnivorous self, see page 233. In the meantime, give yourself 1 point in the Counting Carbs (CCarbs) column. If you have a score of 11 to 20, give yourself 1 point in the Counting Calories (CCals) column. If you have a score of 10 or less, give yourself 1 point in the Counting Fats (CFats) column.

Diet type: CCarbs___ CCals___ CFats___

Dairy Products

7. How often did you drink milk or milk products this week? (For those of you who put milk or cream in your coffee, consider each cup of coffee with milk as ½ serving, so 2 cups are one serving, 4 cups are two servings, and so on.)

   a. Never

   b. 1 to 3 times

   c. 4 to 6 times

   d. 7 or more

7. _____

8. How often did you use butter this week either to cook with or to flavour with?

   a. Never

   b. 1 to 3 times

   c. 4 to 6 times

   d. Daily

   8. _____

9. How often did you eat cheese this week?

   a. Never

   b. 1 to 3 times

   c. 4 to 6 times

   d. Daily

   9. _____

10. How often did you eat yoghurt or ice cream this week?

   a. Never

   b. 1 to 3 times

   c. 4 to 6 times

   d. Daily

   10. _____

Scoring 7 to 10: Give yourself 1 point for every *a*, 5 for every *b*, 10 for every *c*, and 20 for every *d*.

Total: _____

If you have a score greater than 50, then perhaps you are a Dairy Queen/King. For details on how to make your love of all that is dairy work in your diet, see page 243. In the meantime, give yourself 1 point in the Counting Carbs (CCarbs) column and 1 in the Counting Calories (CCals) column. If you have a score of 20 to 50, give yourself 1 point in the Counting Calories column. If you have a score less than 20, give yourself 1 point in the Counting Fats (CFats) column.

Diet type: CCarbs___ CCals___ CFats___

Fruits and Vegetables

11. How often did you eat salad this week?

    a. Never

    b. 1 to 3 times

    c. 4 to 6 times

    d. Daily

    11. _____

12. How often did you eat a green vegetable (not including what was in your salad) this week?

    a. Never

    b. 1 to 3 times

    c. 4 to 6 times

    d. Daily

    12. _____

13. How often did you eat any red, orange, yellow, purple or white vegetables (not including potatoes, which I ask about later, or other veggies in your salad) this week?

    a. Never

    b. 1 to 3 times

    c. 4 to 6 times

    d. Daily

    13. _____

14. How often did you eat fruit this week? (Please count fruit juice as ½ serving.)

    a. Never

    b. 1 to 3 times

    c. 4 to 6 times

    d. Daily

14. _____

Scoring 11 to 14: Give yourself 1 point for every *a*, 5 for every *b*, 10 for every *c*, and 20 for every *d*.

Total: _____

If you have a score greater than 40, perhaps you are a Vegecarian. For details on how to make your love of vegetables work in your diet, see page 247. In the meantime, give yourself 1 point in the Counting Fats (CFats) column. If you have a score of 20 to 40, give yourself 1 point in the Counting Calories (CCals) column. If you have a score less than 20, give yourself 1 point in the Counting Carbs (CCarbs) column.

| Diet type: CCarbs____ CCals____ CFats____ |

Starches

15. How often did you eat potatoes this week?

    a. Never

    b. 1 to 3 times

    c. 4 to 6 times

    d. Daily

15. _____

16. How often did you eat rice this week?

   a. Never

   b. 1 to 3 times

   c. 4 to 6 times

   d. Daily

   16. _____

17. How often did you eat pasta this week?

   a. Never

   b. 1 to 3 times

   c. 4 to 6 times

   d. Daily

   17. _____

18. How often did you eat bread this week? (Count a sandwich as a single serving.)

   a. Never

   b. 1 to 3 times

   c. 4 to 6 times

   d. Daily

   18. _____

19. How often did you eat baked goods other than bread this week? This would include crackers, biscuits, muffins, bagels, cakes and other pastries.

   a. Never

   b. 1 to 3 times

   c. 4 to 6 times

   d. Daily

   19. _____

20. How often did you eat either hot or cold cereal this week?

    a. Never

    b. 1 to 3 times

    c. 4 to 6 times

    d. Daily

20. _____

Scoring 15 to 20: Give yourself 1 point for every *a*, 5 for every *b*, 10 for every *c*, and 20 for every *d*.

Total: _____

If you have a score greater than 40, then perhaps you are a Starch Stealer. For details on how to make your love of starches part of your diet, see page 254. In the meantime, give yourself 1 point in the Counting Fats (CFats) column. If you have a score of 10 to 40, give yourself 1 point in the Counting Calories (CCals) column. If you have a score less than 10, give yourself 1 point in the Counting Carbs (CCarbs) column.

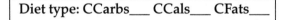

> Diet type: CCarbs___ CCals___ CFats___

Sweets

21. How often did you eat sweet baked goods this week? This would include many of the foods listed in section above: muffins, biscuits, cakes and other pastries.

    a. Never

    b. 1 to 3 times

c. 4 to 6 times

d. Daily

21. _____

22. How often did you eat chocolate this week?

a. Never

b. 1 to 3 times

c. 4 to 6 times

d. Daily

22. _____

23. How often did you eat confectionery other than chocolate this week?

a. Never

b. 1 to 3 times

c. 4 to 6 times

d. Daily

23. _____

24. How often did you drink something sweet this week? This would include soft drinks, sweetened milk drinks and your tea or coffee if you add sweeteners of any sort to it.

a. Never

b. 1 to 3 times

c. 4 to 6 times

d. Daily

24. _____

25. How often did you eat fruit or fruit-based sweets or snacks this week? This would include fruit salad, stewed fruits, dried fruits and foods like that.

a. Never

b. 1 to 3 times

c. 4 to 6 times

d. Daily

25. _____

Scoring 21 to 25: Give yourself 1 point for every *a*, 5 for every *b*, 10 for every *c*, and 20 for every *d*.

Total: _____

If you have a score greater than 40, perhaps you are a Sweets Eater. For details on how to make your love of sweets work in your diet, see page 259. In the meantime, give yourself 1 point in the Counting Fats (CFats) column. If you have a score of 10 to 40, give yourself 1 point in the Counting Calories (CCals) column. If you have a score less than 10, give yourself 1 point in the Counting Carbs (CCarbs) column.

Diet type: CCarbs___ CCals___ CFats___

Liquids

26. How many glasses of water did you drink on average each day during this week?

a. Less than 1 glass per day

b. 1 to 2 glasses per day

c. 3 to 5 glasses per day

d. 6 or more glasses per day

26. _____

27. How many glasses of soft drinks did you have on average each day during this week?

    a. Less than 1 glass per day

    b. 1 to 2 glasses per day

    c. 3 to 5 glasses per day

    d. 6 or more glasses per day

    27. _____

28. How often did you drink fruit juice on average each day during this week?

    a. Less than 1 glass per day

    b. 1 to 2 glasses per day

    c. 3 to 5 glasses per day

    d. 6 or more glasses per day

    28. _____

29. How often did you drink tea or herbal tea on average each day during this week?

    a. Less than 1 glass per day

    b. 1 to 2 glasses per day

    c. 3 to 5 glasses per day

    d. 6 or more glasses per day

    29. _____

30. How often did you drink coffee on average each day during this week?

    a. More than 6 cups a day

    b. 4 to 6 cups per day

    c. 1 to 3 cups per day

    d. Less than 1 cup per day

    30. _____

31. How often did you have a glass of wine or beer or other alcoholic beverage during this week?

   a. More than 4 drinks on 1 or more days this week

   b. 1 to 3 drinks per day

   c. Less than 1 drink per day

   d. None

31. _____

Scoring 26 to 31: Give yourself 1 point for every *a*, 5 for every *b*, 10 for every *c*, and 20 for every *d*.

Total: _____

If you have a score of 30 or less, then perhaps you are a Waterless Wonder – that is, you don't drink enough water. For details on how to work with this aspect of your diet, see page 268. In the meantime, give yourself 1 point in both the Counting Calories (CCals) and Counting Fats (CFats) columns. If you have a score greater than 30, you are pretty well hydrated; give yourself 1 point in the Counting Carbs (CCarbs) column.

Diet type: CCarbs____ CCals____ CFats____

Simplified PROP Test

Answer these questions based on what you know about the way you eat.

32. I find Brussels sprouts:

   a. Very tasty

   b. Moderately tasty

   c. Moderately distasteful

   d. Very distasteful

32. _____

33. I find broccoli:

   a. Very tasty

   b. Moderately tasty

   c. Moderately distasteful

   d. Very distasteful

33. _____

34. I find saccharin:

   a. Very sweet

   b. Moderately sweet

   c. Sweet but somewhat bitter

   d. Sweet but very bitter

34. _____

35. I find grapefruit (without sugar):

   a. Very tasty

   b. Moderately tasty

   c. Moderately distasteful

   d. Very distasteful

35. _____

36. I do not like foods that taste bitter.

   T   F

36. _____

37. I do not like foods that are too sweet.

   T   F

37. _____

38. I do not like foods that are very rich.

   T   F

                                                          38. _____

Scoring 32 to 38: For the multiple choice questions, give yourself 1 point for every *a*, 5 for every *b*, 10 for every *c*, and 20 for every *d*. For the true/false questions, give yourself 0 points for every false and 10 points for every true.

Total for 32 to 38: _____

If you have a score of 40 or greater, you may be a PROP taster. If your score is greater than 80, you may even be a supertaster. For details on this aspect of your eating self, see page 277. In the meantime, give yourself 1 point in the Counting Calories (CCals) column and 1 in the Counting Carbohydrates (CCarbs) column. If your score is less than 50, give yourself 1 point in the Counting Fats (CFats) column.

Diet type: CCarbs___ CCals___ CFats___

DIETING HISTORY

What Makes You Feel Full

39. The most successful diet I have tried was:
    a. Low-fat
    b. Low-calorie

   c. Low-carbohydrate

   d. None of the above

                     39. _____

40. My most common reason for failing on a diet was (pick as many as apply):

   a. A feeling that I hadn't eaten enough

   b. Boredom with the foods I was 'allowed' to eat

   c. Hunger

   d. None of the above

                     40. _____

41. When I'm on a diet, the thing I miss most is (pick as many as apply):

   a. Eating 'enough' to feel full

   b. Eating a variety of foods

   c. Eating rich foods

   d. None of the above

                     41. _____

42. Select any of the following statements about how you eat (pick as many as apply):

   a. What I eat is less important to my satisfaction than how much I eat.

   b. Sometimes when I feel hungry, I find myself standing at the refrigerator door trying to figure out what I am hungry for.

   c. It's very hard for me to feel full unless there is meat or cheese in a meal.

   d. None of the above

                     42. _____

43. Select any of the following statements about how you eat (pick as many as apply):

   a. I don't feel full unless I have eaten a lot of food

   b. I don't feel full unless I have eaten a variety of foods

c. I don't feel full unless I have eaten protein and fat as well as carbohydrates

d. None of the above

43. _____

44. Select any of the following statements about how you eat (pick as many as apply):

a. I could never give up bread, rice or pasta

b. I could never completely give up any category of food

c. I could never become a vegetarian

d. None of the above

44. _____

45. Select any of the following statements about how you eat (pick as many as apply):

a. I could give up meat, so long as I could eat a lot of any other food

b. It's easier for me to restrict my portion size than the type of food I eat

c. I could be happy eating a small variety of foods if I didn't have to restrict my portion size

d. None of the above

45. _____

Scoring 39 to 45: We will score this a little differently. Tally up how many of each letter you picked: *a*'s, *b*'s, *c*'s, *d*'s.

If you picked more than 5 *a*'s, give yourself 1 point in the Counting Fats (CFats) column. Chances are you take your satiety cues from the *volume* of food you eat; you can read about that on page 283.

If you picked *b*'s more than 5 times, give yourself 1 point in the Counting Calories (CCals) column. Your answers suggest that you take your satiety cues from the *variety* of foods you eat. You can read about that on page 288.

If you picked more than 5 *c*'s, then give yourself 1 point in the Counting Carbs (CCarbs) column. Your answers suggest that you take your satiety cues from the *richness* of the foods you eat. You can read more about that on page 291.

If you picked mostly *d*'s, then you have some other satiety cues, and you need to evaluate what makes you full and satisfied. If nothing ever makes you satisfied or full, you should at least consider the possibility that you have an eating disorder. More likely you have cues that I haven't asked about.

Finally, if you ended up evenly divided among two or three categories, you get your satiety cues from more than one of these aspects. Give yourself 1 point in each of the appropriate columns.

Diet type: CCarbs___ CCals___ CFats___

How Dieting Changes the Way You Eat

(If you have never dieted before, you should skip this section.)

46. I have dieted:

    a. Occasionally

    b. Frequently

    c. All the time

46. _____

47. In general, these diets were:

    a. Very successful (I lost weight and kept it all off for greater than 6 months)

    b. Transiently successful (I lost weight but gained it back within 6 months)

    c. Never successful (I never lost any significant weight)

                                               47. _____

48. When I see someone eating something, it often makes me want to eat that, even if I am not hungry.

    a. Never

    b. Once or twice a week

    c. Frequently

                                               48. _____

49. Which statement describes how you feel while dieting?

    a. I sometimes eat less at a meal than I would like to eat

    b. When I have eaten the amount of food I think I should eat, I am pretty good about not eating any more

    c. When I eat something that is not on my diet, it's hard to get back on track

                                               49. _____

50. My weight has changed by more than 9kg (20lb) over the past year. (If you were pregnant in the past year, count the previous year's weight.)

    T   F

                                               50. _____

51. I'm a yo-yo dieter.

    T   F

                                               51. _____

52. When I eat something that is not on my diet, I often find it difficult to resume my diet.

T   F

52. _____

53. When I see someone overeat, I have a tendency to overeat too.

T   F

53. _____

Scoring 46 to 53: For the multiple choice questions, give yourself 1 point for every *a*, 5 for every *b*, and 10 for every *c*. For the true/false questions, give yourself 0 points for every false and 10 points for every true.

Total for 46 to 53: _____

If you have a score greater than 30, then some of your dieting behaviours may be contributing to your inability to manage your weight. For more information on that, see page 295.

Binge Eating Disorder

54. Which of the following responses best describes your overall eating patterns?

   a. I never have trouble with overeating

   b. I sometimes feel that I eat too much during particular eating episodes

   c. I occasionally eat within a 2-hour period what I and most people would consider an unusually large amount of food

d. I quite often eat within a 2-hour period what I and most people would consider an unusually large amount of food.

54. _____

If you answered *a* or *b*, then you are unlikely to have a binge-eating disorder, and you can skip to the next section.

55. When you eat a large amount of food within a 2-hour period, how often do you feel as if you cannot stop eating or control what or how much you eat?

   a. Never

   b. Rarely

   c. Occasionally

   d. Always

55. _____

56. How do you feel when this type of eating takes place? (Pick as many as apply.)

   a. My eating is more rapid than usual

   b. I eat until I feel uncomfortably full

   c. The eating occurs when I am not feeling physically hungry

   d. When I experience this eating behaviour, I do it alone, because I am embarrassed by the amount of food I eat

   e. After my eating episode, I feel disgusted with myself, depressed, or guilty for overeating

56. _____

57. How often have you engaged in this type of behaviour over the past 6 months?

   a. Less than once a month

   b. Once a month to a few times a month

   c. A few times a month to two times a week

d. Two times a week

e. Daily

57. _____

58. When you eat large amounts of food at one time and feel as though you cannot stop eating, how certain are you that you can control these episodes of eating?

a. Extremely certain

b. Quite certain

c. Somewhat certain

d. Slightly certain

e. Not at all certain

58. _____

59. How upset were you that you were not able to control what or how much you were eating?

a. Not at all upset

b. Slightly upset

c. Somewhat upset

d. Quite upset

59. _____

Scoring 54 to 59: Give yourself 1 point for every *a*, 2 for every *b*, 3 for every *c*, 4 for every *d*, and 5 for every *e*.

Total: _____

If your score is less than 11, you are not likely to have an eating disorder. If your score is 11 or higher, you are at risk of having one and should discuss this with your doctor before starting on any diet. (See page 296 for more information.)

MEDICAL HISTORY

Your Own History

60. I smoke cigarettes.

   T   F

   60. _____

61. I have high total cholesterol (above 5.0 mmol/L).

   T   F   Never tested

   61. _____

62. I have high LDL cholesterol (above 3.0 mmol/L).

   T   F   Never tested

   62. _____

63. I have low HDL cholesterol (below 1.1 mmol/L).

   T   F   Never tested

   63. _____

64. I have high triglycerides (2.0 mmol/L or above).

   T   F   Never tested

   64. _____

65. My doctor has prescribed medicine for my cholesterol.

   T   F

   65. _____

66. I have diabetes.

   T   F

   66. _____

67. I take medicine for diabetes.

    T   F

                                             67. _____

68. I have high blood pressure (greater than 140/90 mm Hg).

    T   F   Never tested

                                             68. _____

69. I take medicine for high blood pressure.

    T   F

                                             69. _____

70. I have heart disease (angina, coronary artery disease, history of heart attack).

    T   F

                                             70. _____

71. My doctor has prescribed medicine for my heart disease.

    T   F

                                             71. _____

Scoring 60 to 71: Give yourself 1 point for every true and 0 points for every false.

Total: _____

If you are under the age of 30 and marked any of the questions 'Never tested', count those as 0 and continue. If you are over the age of 30 and marked any of the questions 'Never tested', you should contact your doctor for further evaluation of your cardiac risk factors.

If you are a man, give yourself an extra point. If you are a man and over 55, give yourself another extra point. If you are a woman and you are past menopause, give yourself an extra point.

Total: _____

If you have a score of 3 or greater, chances are that you are at increased risk of heart disease and should consult your doctor before starting any diet or exercise regime. For further information on what these cardiac risk factors mean, turn to page 299. If you have a score of 3 or greater, give yourself 1 point in the Counting Fats (CFats) column. If you have a score ranging from 0 to 2, give yourself 1 point in both the Counting Carbohydrates (CCarbs) and Counting Calories (CCals) columns.

Diet type: CCarbs___ CCals___ CFats___

Family History

72. My father had a heart attack before he was 45.

   T   F   Don't know

72. _____

73. My mother had a heart attack before she was 55.

   T   F   Don't know

73. _____

74. My mother or father has had coronary bypass surgery.

   T   F   Don't know

74. _____

75. My mother or father has diabetes.

   T   F   Don't know

                                                    75. _____

76. My mother or father has high blood pressure.

   T   F   Don't know

                                                    76. _____

77. My mother or father has high cholesterol.

   T   F   Don't know

                                                    77. _____

   Scoring 72 to 77: Give yourself 1 point for every true and 0 points for every false.

Total: _____

   These are also cardiac risk factors. If you answered true on two of these questions, you should consult your doctor before starting any diet and exercise regime. For more information on what these risk factors mean, turn to page 312. If you can't find out your parents' medical history, you can skip this section. If you only know one parent's medical history, then double the points and follow the directions based on that. If you have a score of 3 or greater, give yourself 1 point in the Counting Fats (CFats) column. If you have a score ranging from 0 to 2, give yourself 1 point in both the Counting Carbohydrates (CCarbs) and Counting Calories (CCals) columns.

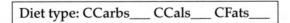

Diet type: CCarbs____ CCals____ CFats____

78. I have low HDL cholesterol (below 1.0 mmol/L for men and below 1.1 mmol/L for women).

    T   F   Never tested

                             78. _____

79. I have high triglycerides (2.0 mmol/L or above).

    T   F   Never tested

                             79. _____

80. I carry much of my extra weight around my middle (waist 102cm/40in or greater for men; 88cm/35in or greater for women).

    T   F   Never tested (so test it now)

                             80. _____

81. I have high blood pressure or am taking medicine for high blood pressure.

    T   F   Never tested (so get it tested now)

                             81. _____

82. I have diabetes or am taking medicine for diabetes.

    T   F   Never tested

                             82. _____

Scoring 78 to 82: Give yourself 1 point for every true and 0 points for every false.

Total: _____

If you have a score of 3 or more, you have metabolic syndrome, and you can read about what this means in terms of how you should eat on page 309. Also give yourself 2 points in the Counting Carbohydrates (CCarbs) column and 1 point in the Counting Calories (CCals) column. If you answered true to two questions and don't know your HDL cholesterol or your triglycerides or haven't been tested for diabetes, you should discuss your risk with your doctor and ask him to test you for metabolic syndrome. If you have a score greater than 0 but less than 3, you do not have metabolic syndrome, but you are at risk of developing it. You also should read about this condition and the diet that can lower your risk of developing the condition. Also give yourself 1 point in the Counting Calories (CCals) column. If you have a score of 0, then give yourself 1 point in the Counting Fats (CFats) column.

> Diet type: CCarbs___ CCals___ CFats___

FAMILY HERITAGE

How You Are Shaped by Nature

83. In my family (mark all that apply):
    a. I am not overweight
    b. I am the only one who is overweight
    c. My mother is overweight
    d. My father is overweight
    e. One or more of my siblings are overweight
    f. All of my siblings are overweight

    83. _____

84. I am overweight in the same way as my (mark all that apply):
    a. I am not overweight
    b. Mother

c. Father

d. Siblings

e. Grandparents

f. None of the above

84. _____

85. I have a lot of nervous energy and need to move almost all the time.

T   F

85. _____

86. One or both of my parents have a lot of nervous energy and need to move almost all the time.

T   F

86. _____

87. No one in my family likes vegetables.

T   F

87. _____

88. Everyone in my family likes meat.

T   F

88. _____

89. When I see someone overeating, I am more likely to overeat as well.

T   F

89. _____

90. I have noticed that others in my family overeat when they are around someone who is overeating.

T   F

90. _____

Scoring 83 to 90: Give yourself 1 point for every marked answer in the multiple choice questions. For the true/false questions, give yourself 1 point for every true answer and 0 points for every false.

Total: _____

If you have a score of 4 or less, then genetics are not playing an important role in your weight. If you have a score of 5 or more, genetics are probably playing an important role in your weight. For more information on how your genes can affect your weight, see page 315.

How You Are Shaped by Nurture

91. When I was growing up, food was used as a reward.

    T   F

                                          91. _____

92. When I was growing up, food was used as a form of medicine for physical or emotional injuries.

    T   F

                                          92. _____

93. When I was growing up, the meals I ate with my family were the best part of a day.

    T   F

                                          93. _____

94. When I was growing up, cleaning your plate was a must at the dinner table.

    T   F

                                          94. _____

95. When I was growing up, meals were characterized by:

   a. Just the right amount of food

   b. Too much food

   c. Too little food

   d. Occasions when members of my family went hungry because there wasn't enough food.

                                   95. _____

96. When I was growing up:

   a. My family frequently engaged in sports or other physical activities together (hiking, cycling, gardening, etc.)

   b. My family occasionally engaged in sports or other physical activities together

   c. My parents weren't active but encouraged and helped me participate in sports or other physical activities

   d. My parents discouraged my participation in sports or other physical activities

                                   96. _____

97. When I was growing up:

   a. I was always involved in sports and other physical activities

   b. I frequently participated in sports or other physical activities

   c. I occasionally participated in sports or other physical activities

   d. I rarely participated in sports or other physical activities

                                   97. _____

98. When I was growing up:

   a. I watched television less than 4 hours per week

   b. I watched television between 4 and 8 hours per week

c. I watched television between 8 and 12 hours per week

d. I watched television more than 12 hours per week

98. _____

Scoring 91 to 98: For true/false questions, give yourself 1 point for every true and 0 points for every false. For multiple choice questions, give yourself 0 points for every *a*, 1 for every *b*, 5 for every *c*, and 10 for every *d*.

Total: _____

If you have a score of 15 or more, your experiences growing up may be contributing to your difficulty managing your weight now. For more information on this, turn to page 319.

HOW YOU EAT

Eating Habits

99. I skip breakfast:

   a. Never or rarely

   b. Once or twice a week

   c. Several times a week

   d. I always skip breakfast

99. _____

100. I skip lunch:

   a. Never or rarely

   b. Once or twice a week

    c. Several times a week

    d. I always skip lunch

100. _____

101. I skip dinner:

    a. Never or rarely

    b. Once or twice a week

    c. Several times a week

    d. I always skip dinner

101. _____

102. When I sit down to a meal, I feel like I'm starving:

    a. Never or rarely

    b. One or two meals per week

    c. Most meals

    d. Every meal

102. _____

103. I snack before lunch:

    a. Never or rarely

    b. Once or twice a week

    c. Several times a week

    d. Most days

103. _____

104. I snack between lunch and dinner:

    a. Never or rarely

    b. Once or twice a week

    c. Several times a week

    d. Most days

104. _____

105. I snack after dinner:

    a. Never or rarely

    b. Once or twice a week

    c. Several times a week

    d. Most days

                                             105. _____

106. I am so hungry at some point during the day that I feel as if I have to eat something right away:

    a. Never or rarely

    b. Once or twice a week

    c. Several times a week

    d. Most days

                                           106. _____

Scoring 99 to 106: Give yourself 1 point for every *a*, 5 for every *b*, 10 for every *c*, and 20 for every *d*.

Total: _____

If you have a score of less than 10, then you have pretty good eating habits, and the foods you eat are keeping you full from meal to meal. If you have a score of 10 to 40, your eating habits may be contributing to your difficulty achieving and maintaining your target weight. If you have a score greater than 40, then how you structure your eating is very likely contributing to your difficulty in achieving and maintaining your target weight. For information on what we know about effective eating habits, see page 322.

Emotional Eating

Answer these questions based on your diet diary as well as on what you know about yourself.

107. I eat because of boredom:
    a. Never
    b. Occasionally, but never more than once a week
    c. Frequently – at least twice a week
    d. Daily

    107. _____

108. I eat because I feel stressed:
    a. Never
    b. Occasionally, but never more than once a week
    c. Frequently – at least twice a week
    d. Daily

    108. _____

109. I eat because of an unpleasant emotion, such as anger or depression:
    a. Never
    b. Occasionally, but never more than once a week
    c. Frequently – at least twice a week
    d. Daily

    109. _____

110. I eat as a reward:
    a. Never
    b. Occasionally, but never more than once a week
    c. Frequently – at least twice a week
    d. Daily

    110. _____

111. I eat for comfort:

a. Never

b. Occasionally, but never more than once a week

c. Frequently – at least twice a week

d. Daily

111. _____

112. I eat while watching television:

a. Never

b. Occasionally, but never more than once a week

c. Frequently – at least twice a week

d. Daily

112. _____

113. I eat while engaged in another activity, such as reading or driving:

a. Never

b. Occasionally, but never more than once a week

c. Frequently – at least twice a week

d. Daily

113. _____

Scoring 107 to 113: Give yourself 1 point for every *a*, 5 for every *b*, 10 for every *c*, and 20 for every *d*.

Total: _____

If your score is less than 15, you have pretty good eating habits and usually do not use food to address a non-hunger need. Good for you. If you have a score of 15 to 40, then emotional eating may be contributing to your difficulty achieving and maintaining your target weight. If your score is greater than 40, emotional eating is very likely contributing to your difficulty achieving and maintaining your target weight. To learn about emotional eating, see page 330.

LIFESTYLE

Eating Out

Some of these answers draw on your food diary.

114. In my food diary, I ate out at a restaurant:

a. Never or rarely

b. Once

c. 2 to 4 times

d. More than 4 times

114. _____

115. In an average week, I eat out:

a. Never or rarely

b. Once

c. 2 to 4 times

d. More than 4 times

115. _____

116. In an average week, I am most likely to stop at a fast-food restaurant for a meal:

a. Never or rarely

b. Once

c. 2 to 4 times

d. More than 4 times

116. _____

117. In my food diary, I ate while at my desk:

   a. Never or rarely

   b. Once

   c. 2 to 4 times

   d. More than 4 times

   117. _____

118. In my food diary, I ate while driving or in a parked car:

   a. Never or rarely

   b. Once

   c. 2 to 4 times

   d. More than 4 times

   118. _____

Scoring 114 to 118: Give yourself 1 point for every *a*, 5 for every *b*, 10 for every *c*, and 20 for every *d*.

Total: _____

In you have a score of 20 or more, where you are eating may be having a big impact on your ability to lose weight or maintain your weight loss. Turn to page 338 for some tips on how to work with these common problems of modern life. If you have more than 40 points, you eat out a lot, so give yourself 1 point in the Counting Carbohydrates (CCarbs) column. If you have a score of less than 20, then chances are you are in pretty good control of what you eat, so give yourself 1 point in each of the three diet columns. If you scored 20 to 40 points, you eat out of the house often enough so that a diet that requires you to keep track of fat will be useless. Give yourself

1 point in the Counting Carbohydrates (CCarbs) column and in the Counting Calories (CCals) column.

| Diet type: CCarbs____ CCals____ CFats____ |

Daily Activity

Answer these questions based on your activity diary.

119. Most days, I climbed stairs:

    a. Never or rarely

    b. 1 or 2 flights per day

    c. 3 to 5 flights per day

    d. More than 5 flights per day

                                                119. _____

120. Most days I walked:

    a. no more than 400m ($\frac{1}{4}$ mile)

    b. 400–800m ($\frac{1}{4}$–$\frac{1}{2}$ mile)

    c. 800m ($\frac{1}{2}$ mile)

    d. More than 2km ($1\frac{1}{4}$ miles)

                                                120. _____

121. Which best describes how you got to your workplace?

    a. I drove to work and parked nearby

    b. I drove to work, parked and walked a block or so to work

    c. I took public transport to work

    d. I walked or cycled to work

                                                121. _____

122. Which best describes how much time you spent sitting (both at work and at home)?

    a. I sat more than 12 hours per day

    b. I sat between 8 and 12 hours per day

    c. I sat between 4 and 8 hours per day

    d. I sat less than 4 hours per day

                                                122. _____

123. Which best describes how much time per week you spent doing housework (cleaning, cooking, laundry, etc.)?

    a. Less than 1 hour per week

    b. Between 1 and 3 hours per week

    c. Between 3 and 6 hours per week

    d. More than 6 hours per week

                                                123. _____

124. Which best describes how much time per week you spent working in your garden?

    a. Are you kidding? Who has the time or the space for a garden?

    b. Less than 2 hours per week

    c. Between 2 and 5 hours per week

    d. More than 5 hours per week

                                                124. _____

125. Which best describes how much time each day you spent watching television?

    a. More than 5 hours per day

    b. Between 3 and 5 hours per day

    c. Between 1 and 3 hours per day

    d. Less than 1 hour per day

                                                125. _____

126. Which best describes how much time each day you spent in your car?

    a. More than 5 hours per day

    b. Between 3 and 5 hours per day

    c. Between 1 and 3 hours per day

    d. Less than 1 hour per day

126. _____

127. Which best describes how much time each day you spent exercising?

    a. Are you kidding? Who has time to exercise?

    b. Between 5 minutes and a half an hour

    c. Between a half an hour to an hour

    d. More than 1 hour

127. _____

128. Most weeks I work outside the home (include volunteer work as well as work for which you are paid):

    a. Greater than 50 hours per week

    b. Between 40 and 50 hours per week

    c. Between 25 and 40 hours per week

    d. Less than 25 hours per week

128. _____

Scoring 119 to 128: Give yourself 1 point for every *a*, 5 for every *b*, 10 for every *c*, and 20 for every *d*.

Total: _____

If you have a score of 45 or less, chances are your lifestyle and activity level contribute to your difficulty in losing weight or maintaining your weight loss. Turn to page 344 to learn more about how normal daily activity can contribute to your effort to control your weight.

Exercise

129. I have so many responsibilities that I don't have time for myself.

    T   F

    129. _____

130. I don't have any friends who exercise.

    T   F

    130. _____

131. Most people I know are overweight.

    T   F

    131. _____

132. I am too busy to exercise.

    T   F

    132. _____

133. I don't enjoy exercise.

    T   F

    133. _____

134. There is no place for me to exercise.

    T   F

    134. _____

135. I hate working out in gyms.

    T   F

    135. _____

136. I'm uncomfortable in a gym because of how I look.

    T   F

    136. _____

137. I have never been in good shape.

    T   F

    137. _____

138. I have never exercised regularly.

T   F

138. _____

139. I feel silly or incompetent when I exercise.

T   F

139. _____

140. I live in an urban environment where it is hard to exercise outside.

T   F

140. _____

141. Most weeks I exercise:

a. More than 4 times

b. 3 to 4 times

c. Once or twice

d. Never

141. _____

Scoring 129 to 141: Give yourself 0 points for every false, 1 point for every true, 1 point for every *a*, 5 points for *b*, 10 points for *c*, and 20 points for *d*.

Total: _____

If you scored more than 10 points, you have some serious resistance to exercise. If you scored 5 to 10, you have a good attitude towards exercise but probably need to increase the frequency. This may be a time issue or this may be a pleasure issue. For help figuring out how to get past these problems, check out page 348. If you scored below 5, congratulations! You have a good attitude to exercise, and you do it regularly.

SCORING THE QUESTIONNAIRE

Now is the time when we tally up all the diet preferences and see which one is right for you.

Count up all the points you put in the Counting Carbohydrates, Counting Calories and Counting Fats columns.

Counting Carbohydrates Diet (CCarbs): ___
Counting Calories Diet (CCals): ___
Counting Fats Diet (CFats): ___

The maximum number of points you could get in any single diet is 13. The diet that gets the most points is the diet for you. You should go to the chapter on that type of diet and read up on it. For example, if you scored highest in the Counting Fats column, then turn to chapter 8 and read up on the whys and wherefores of counting fats. If instead you scored most in the Counting Carbs column, then turn to chapter 6.

Each diet chapter starts with the big picture of the diet – what you should be eating and why. There is also a list of foods in serving sizes that are calculated in the scale that is appropriate for your diet. For example, the Counting Carbs plan has a list of foods in quantities that have less than 5 grams of carbohydrates. Lastly, you will find a 7-day eating plan to give you some guidance as to how to put these foods together to make an actual diet. These are diets that I developed based on the research I have done in nutrition.

What if you ended up evenly split between two diet varieties? There is a maximum of 13 points, and it's possible for someone to score 5 and 5 and 3 and be completely confused. In that case, you should go one extra step: the first seven sections, questions 1 to 38, are the questions that look at food preferences. Which plan gets the highest score there? (If there was a tie, count both.)

Food Preferences score: Diet type: CCarbs___ CCals___ CFats___

Next, look at questions 39 to 45 in the Dieting History section, and write down which plan gets the highest score there. (Again, if there was a tie, count both.)

Diet History score: Diet type: CCarbs___ CCals___ CFats___

Third, look at questions 60 to 71 in the Medical History section, and write down which plan gets the highest score there.

Medical History score: Diet type: CCarbs___ CCals___ CFats___

Then, look at the section on Metabolic Syndrome, questions 78 to 82, and write down which plan gets the highest score there.

Metabolic Syndrome score: Diet type: CCarbs___ CCals___ CFats___

Finally, look at the section on Eating Out, questions 114 through 118, and mark which plan gets the highest score there.

Eating Out score: Diet type: CCarbs___ CCals___ CFats___

Whichever one of those gets 3 out of 5 points is the plan most likely to fit you perfectly. Now let's get started.

THE ANSWER PAGE

Use this page to keep track of your answers so you can tally them up.

FOOD PREFERENCES

Meat and Eggs

1. ____   4. ____   Total for 1 to 6: ____

2. ____   5. ____   Diet type: CCarbs___ CCals___ CFats___

3. ____   6. ____   Are you a Carnimore? If so, see page 233.

Dairy Products

7. ____   9. ____   Total for 7 to 10: ____

8. ____   10. ____   Diet type: CCarbs___ CCals___ CFats___

Are you a Dairy Queen/King? If so, see page 243.

Fruits and Vegetables

11. ____   13. ____   Total for 11 to 14: ____

12. ____   14. ____   Diet type: CCarbs___ CCals___ CFats___

Are you a Vegecarian? If so, see page 247.

Starches

15. ____   18. ____   Total for 15 to 20: ____

16. ____   19. ____   Diet type: CCarbs___ CCals___ CFats___

17. ____   20. ____   Are you a Starch Stealer? If so, see page 254.

Sweets

21. ____   24. ____   Total for 21 to 25: ____

22. ____   25. ____   Diet type: CCarbs___ CCals___ CFats___

23. ____   Are you a Sweets Eater? If so, see page 259.

Liquids

26. _____   29. _____   Total for 26 to 31: _____

27. _____   30. _____   Diet type: CCarbs___ CCals___ CFats___

28. _____   31. _____   Are you a Waterless Wonder? If so, see page 268.

Simplified PROP Test

32. _____   36. _____   Total for 32 to 38: _____

33. _____   37. _____   Diet type: CCarbs___ CCals___ CFats___

34. _____   38. _____   Are you a PROP taster or supertaster? If so, see page 277.

35. _____

DIETING HISTORY

What Makes You Feel Full

39. _____   43. _____   Total for 39 to 45: a's _____ b's _____ c's _____ d's _____

40. _____   44. _____

41. _____   45. _____   Diet type: CCarbs___ CCals___ CFats___

42. _____

Are you satisfied by volume (mostly a's)? If yes, see page 283.

Are you satisfied by variety (mostly b's)? If yes, see page 288.

Are you satisfied by richness (mostly c's)? If yes, see page 291.

How Dieting Changes the Way You Eat

46. _____   50. _____   Total for 46 to 53: _____

47. _____   51. _____   Has dieting affected the way you eat? If so, see page 295.

48. _____   52. _____

49. _____   53. _____

Binge Eating Disorder

54. _____   57. _____   Total for 54 to 59: _____

55. _____   58. _____   Do you have, or are you at risk of, an eating

56. _____   59. _____   disorder? If so, see page 296.

MEDICAL HISTORY

Your Own History

60. _____   66. _____   Total for 60 to 71: _____

61. _____   67. _____   Extra point(s): _____

62. _____   68. _____   Total: _____

63. _____   69. _____   Diet type: CCarbs___ CCals___ CFats___

64. _____   70. _____   Do you have significant risk factors? If so,

65. _____   71. _____   see page 299.

Family History

72. _____   75. _____   Total for 72 to 77: _____

73. _____   76. _____   Diet type: CCarbs___ CCals___ CFats___

74. _____   77. _____   Have you inherited risk factors? If so,
see page 312.

Metabolic Syndrome

78. _____   81. _____   Total for 78 to 82: _____

79. _____   82. _____   Diet type: CCarbs___ CCals___ CFats___

80. _____   Do you have metabolic syndrome? If so, see
page 309.

FAMILY HERITAGE

How You Are Shaped by Nature

83. _____   87. _____   Total for 83 to 90: _____

84. _____   88. _____   Is your genetic makeup playing a role in

85. _____   89. _____   your weight? If so, see page 315.

86. _____   90. _____

How You Are Shaped by Nurture

91. _____   95. _____   Total for 91 to 98: _____

92. _____   96. _____   Are your experiences growing up playing a

93. _____   97. _____   role in your weight? If so, see page 319.

94. _____   98. _____

HOW YOU EAT

Eating Habits

99. _____   103. _____   Total for 99 to 106: _____

100. _____   104. _____   Are your eating habits playing a role in your

101. _____   105. _____   weight? If so, see page 322.

102. _____   106. _____

Emotional Eating

107. _____   111. _____   Total for 107 to 113: _____

108. _____   112. _____   Do you eat to address a non-hunger need?

109. _____   113. _____   If so, see page 330.

110. _____

LIFESTYLE

Eating Out

114. _____   117. _____   Total for 114 to 118: _____

115. _____   118. _____   Diet type: CCarbs___ CCals___ CFats___

116. _____

Does eating away from home contribute to your weight? If so, turn to page 338.

Daily Activity

119. _____   124. _____   Total for 119 to 128: _____

120. _____   125. _____

121. _____   126. _____   Does your activity level contribute to your weight? If so, turn to page 344.

122. _____   127. _____

123. _____   128. _____

Exercise

129. _____   136. _____   Total for 129 to 141: _____

130. _____   137. _____

131. _____   138. _____   Do you have a resistance to exercise, or do you need to exercise more frequently? If so, turn to page 348.

132. _____   139. _____

133. _____   140. _____

134. _____   141. _____

135. _____

PART

THE PERFECT FIT BASIC DIETS

NOW THAT YOU'VE KEPT A WEEK-LONG EATING and exercise diary, and answered and scored your questionnaire, you know a lot more about what, how and why you enjoy certain foods. And you've probably figured out which of the three basic diets is the best fit for you: the Counting Carbohydrates Diet, the Counting Calories Diet or the Counting Fats Diet.

In part 3, I'll take you through each basic diet and explain:

- Why it's likely to be the best weight-loss strategy for you
- The essential principles of the diet as well as what the most up-to-date research has to say about why and how you'll lose weight on this diet
- How to make this kind of diet work for you, so you can reach and maintain your desired weight

At the end of each chapter, I'll also give you a list of foods that are allowed on each diet and offer you a week-long meal plan that can be modified from week to week.

You need to read only the chapter about the basic diet you've been paired with, but if you're still not sure which diet is the best fit for you, then you may want to read about all three of them.

I have created versions of these three basic diet plans based on my research in nutrition and experiences with my own patients. They're similar to other diets in the same category but with unique twists to make them the most effective, the most easily maintained and the safest version of each diet. Essentially, each of them emphasizes foods that are as fresh and unprocessed as possible with a low saturated-fat content and a low glycaemic load. (If any of these terms are unfamiliar to you now, trust me, they won't be by the time you're done selecting and customizing your diet.)

In part 4, I'll show you how to tailor your basic diet to fit your food preferences, medical history and lifestyle to a T. But right now, our job is to give you a chance to familiarize yourself with how your basic diet will work to help you find and maintain your desired weight.

6 CHAPTER

THE COUNTING CARBOHYDRATES DIET

I
T HAS BEEN HAILED AS a 'diet revolution', but it's really been more like the world's oldest food fight. While the low-carbohydrate diet has been around for almost 2,000 years, it got its most recent start in 1972 with the publication of *Dr Atkins' Diet Revolution* by Manhattan-based cardiologist Robert Atkins, MD. That book and its successor, *Dr Atkins' New Diet Revolution*, have triggered a true revolution in diet strategy. Along with Atkins have come a slew of other low-carb diets: the Scarsdale diet, the Zone diet, Protein Power, Suzanne Somers's *Get Skinny on Fabulous Food*, and most recently, the South Beach diet. All maintain that the reason we are fat – and getting fatter – is that we eat too many carbohydrates and carbs make us fat.

Traditional medicine has recoiled in horror at the notion of a diet heavy on meats (and fat) and skimpy on fruits, vegetables and breads. It seemed clear that such a diet would be unhealthy and increase the risk of heart disease and other health problems. The truth is that although this diet runs counter to many of the ideas cherished by several generations of doctors, recent studies show that it is a safe and effective choice for many dieters.

In this chapter we will look first at who does well on this diet. Then I'm going to take you through the basic principles of a low-carbohydrate diet – if you have a grip on how this diet works, you will be able to make it work better for you. We'll briefly review what we know, and don't know, about its safety. The Perfect Fit Counting Carbohydrates Diet is described in detail in the next section, followed by a list of no- and low-carbohydrate foods and a 7-day eating plan. At the end of the chapter, you'll find some recipes that will help you stay within the guidelines of this diet.

There are aspects of this diet that definitely make losing weight easier for some people. First of all, you will be eating very filling and satisfying foods. And you will be avoiding many of the foods that seem to be easy to overeat, such as bread, crisps and sweets. On this diet, you will never feel deprived. While your choice of foods in this diet is the most limited of all the diets, the foods you are allowed to eat are some of the richest, most luxurious foods available.

LINDA'S STORY

Linda is an estate agent who came to see me on the eve of her 39th birthday. It was going to be a year of big changes in her life: she was selling the house she'd had for 20 years, and she and her longtime partner had decided to buy a house together. Next year they were getting married. In spite of, or maybe because of, all these transitions, Linda thought it would be a good time to once again try to get her weight under control.

She was a beautiful woman with a mass of curly brown hair and deep blue eyes. A hint of laugh lines appeared when she smiled – which was often. She told her story briefly: she'd been a 'good size' – not too big, not too small – most of her life. During an unhappy marriage, she became depressed and started putting on weight. Both her parents were heavy, so she would periodically diet to try to sidestep what she increasingly worried was her own fate. But after the kids were born, she just gave up, and the weight accumulated as the years went by. After her divorce, she lost much of her weight, but in the last 5 years she'd started putting it all back on.

She'd tried just about everything: a low-fat diet left her hungry; rotation diets were too hard to follow and were, she thought, rather silly; a low-carbohydrate diet had worked for a while, but after a few months she simply couldn't stand the monotony and gave up on it. Her doctor was concerned about the diet anyway, because her cholesterol was abnormal. She'd even tried one of those weight-loss medications, and though it had worked for a while, she became concerned about the possible health risks and stopped taking it. The weight reappeared like magic.

'I don't know what you can do that I haven't already done, but I feel as if I need to lose this weight now, and I don't know what else to try,' she told me when we met. She filled out the diet diary and the questionnaire.

She was accustomed to eating three meals a day, every day. 'I couldn't skip breakfast or lunch – that's when I'm the hungriest,' she said. When she ate out, which was often (four nights the week of her diary), her usual meal was a salmon steak and a salad. She drank two or three glasses of wine most nights. She rarely ate pasta or sweets, but she loved fruits and vegetables.

She belonged to a gym and worked out regularly when she felt good about herself. These days those trips to the gym were few and far between. She'd worked out only once during the week she kept her activity diary.

After reviewing her diet, her lifestyle and her history, I thought it was clear that Linda would do best on a low-carbohydrate diet. Why? Firstly, of course, her food preferences made this an obvious choice: she ate meat, eggs and cheese almost every day; salads were regular fare for her; and although she ate fruits and vegetables frequently, the starchy carbohydrates that make up so much of a low-fat diet were absent.

Her diet history also pointed towards a low-carb diet. She'd been on a low-fat diet but couldn't stick to it because it was difficult for her to feel full when she just ate salad, no matter how large it was. Plus, a low-fat diet prohibited too many of the foods she loved. Giving up cheese and butter, steak and salmon, passing on the occasional taste of pâté or nuts, made her feel deprived and depressed. She described the resentment she regularly felt at going to a restaurant and ordering a salad while those around her chose the foods that she really wanted.

And the low-carb diet she'd been on seemed to satisfy her – at least initially. Variety wasn't a big issue for her. According to her diary, she'd eaten almost the same meals several times over the course of a week. Although she'd eventually stopped the low-carb diet because of boredom with the food choices, she'd done well on it for several months.

And there was something else too. I asked Linda about her avoidance of pasta. She just shuddered. 'I love pasta, but I can't eat it in moderation, so I just try not to eat it at all. I think I'm addicted to carbs.' A plate of spaghetti or lasagne would send her into a binge of eating that was hard to stop, she reported. Same with sweets, crisps, even popcorn. 'I just can't eat it.'

Linda was a classic carb-counting dieter. She loved the rich foods that make up so much of that diet. She craved them for the satisfaction she felt after eating them and felt deprived and hungry when these foods were off-limits. Because of the very restrictive nature of the low-carb diet, those who do well on this diet do not crave variety or quantity as much as other eaters and can be satisfied by eating a pretty limited palette of very good foods. Although Linda's doctor was worried about her cholesterol, it was her HDL (good) cholesterol and triglycerides that were off, so eating a diet high in carbohydrates (even if she'd trusted herself to eat such a diet) would only make those problems worse. If you find yourself identifying with Linda, chances are that you are a carb counter as well.

THE ATKINS DIET

While carbohydrate-restricted diets have cycled in popularity since the Greek Olympians first used it to power them to victory, Dr Atkins was behind their most recent resurrection. He'd first read about the low-carbohydrate diet in the *Journal of the American Medical Association* in 1963. It came as a revelation to a man desperate for answers for his own weight dilemma.

He describes this discovery in his 1972 book, *Dr Atkins' Diet Revolution*. He was in his early forties and had put on so much weight that he didn't recognize himself in his own ID picture. He knew he had to lose weight but could not imagine dieting. He writes, 'I knew I could never follow a low-calorie diet for even one day . . . I have a big appetite, but I have very little willpower. . . . Even the idea of hunger scares me.' So when he read a study by a researcher in Atlanta who was investigating the metabolic consequences of eliminating carbohydrates from the diet and noted that participants lost an average of 9.1kg (22lb) in 3½ months eating only protein and fat, he was intrigued.

He decided to conduct an experiment – on himself. 'When I started being my own guinea pig, I knew I was going to eat a lot of food and felt that I would be lucky to lose three or four pounds in a month. I was truly surprised – in fact it was probably the greatest surprise of my life – when at the end of six weeks on this diet I had lost twenty-eight pounds!' Thus was born the Atkins diet.

The low-carbohydrate diets designed by Dr Atkins and others turn the traditional Dietary Pyramid – devised by the US Department of Agriculture and adopted by many other countries – on its head, almost literally. In the USDA food pyramid, the widest tiers of the pyramid are occupied by carbohydrates – fruits and vegetables, breads and pastas. It is therefore recommending up to 20 servings of carbs *each day*. At the top of the pyramid in the category 'Use sparingly,' are listed fats, oils and sweets. Below that, the traditional pyramid recommends only 2 to 3 tiny servings of meats and dairy products per day. If you flip this over you get a pretty good picture of the food pyramid as envisioned by low-carbohydrate-diet promoters.

Traditional Food Pyramid

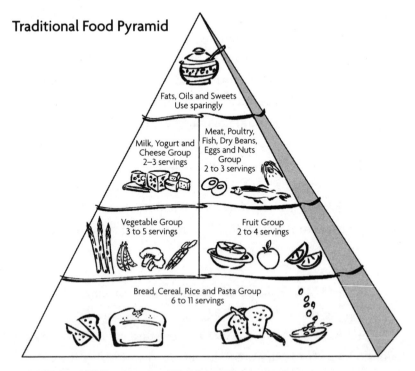

© USDA and US Department of Health and Human Services

THE BASICS
OF A LOW-CARBOHYDRATE DIET

How can this diet, so contrary to traditional low-calorie, low-fat thinking about weight loss and diet, work? Firstly, despite the sales rap, a low-carbohydrate diet *is* a low-calorie diet. The carbohydrates it prohibits are the most abundant foods in the Western diet; up to 60 per cent of our calories each day come from these foods. Eliminate them and chances are you will be taking in far fewer calories, even if you eat more of the foods you're allowed.

Moreover, despite the apparent differences, both the low-fat and low-carbohydrate diets share one important characteristic: the foods prohibited on both these diets are some of the most fattening foods in the marketplace. Which foods? The high-fat, high-carbohydrate foods that have taken an increasingly large role in our diets: crisps,

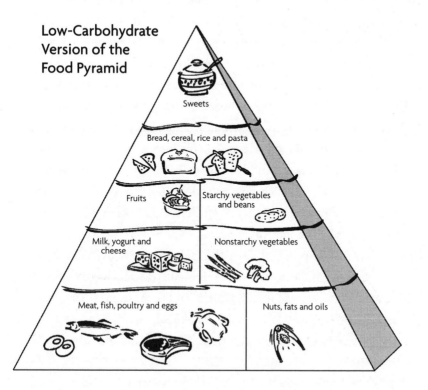

Low-Carbohydrate
Version of the
Food Pyramid

Sweets

Bread, cereal, rice and pasta

Fruits

Starchy vegetables
and beans

Milk, yogurt and
cheese

Nonstarchy vegetables

Meat, fish, poultry and eggs

Nuts, fats and oils

biscuits, cakes and pastries. While coming at these foods from oppo-site directions, both diets eliminate many of the same high-calorie, low-nutritional-value foods.

And the foods remaining in the diet, proteins and fats, are some of the most filling foods we eat. While it's possible – even easy – to consume loads of crisps, overeating high-protein, high-fat foods like steak or creamy sauces is more difficult. They make you too full. Sure, we do it every Christmas, but the overstuffed feeling we get after-wards is enough to remind us not to do it again – at least not for another year. Moreover, the extremely limited variety of food choices available to low-carb dieters helps curb appetite. If, as the saying goes, 'new meat begets new appetite', a diet made up only of meat (and eggs and salad) clearly dampens it.

Hard to believe? But it's true. In studies comparing people on a diet that restricts carbohydrates to those on a low-fat diet, the low-carb group took in fewer calories than the low-fat dieters.

Also, by limiting carbohydrates, you reduce the amount of insulin in your system. And high levels of insulin promote obesity in at least some of us. While low-carbohydrate-diet advocates have said this all along, only recently has science been able to support this theory.

Finally, there is the almost instant weight loss seen in the low-carb diet. One of the first dieters to promote the low-carb diet, 18th-century cabinet maker William Banting, spoke glowingly of the immediate results he saw. 'The great charms and comfort of the system', he noted in a now famous letter, 'are that its effects are palpable within a week of trial and creates a natural stimulus to persevere for a few weeks more'. The diet helped him lose 21kg (46lb) of his 92kg (202lb) in the course of a year, at the age of 66. Traditionally, doctors have scoffed at this claim – not because it isn't true; even the most hard-core critics acknowledge this fact: low-carbohydrate dieters will lose several kilo-grams in the first few days of this diet. Why? Because by eating a diet with virtually no carbohydrates in it, low-carb dieters get rid of the sugar stored in the liver (glycogen) within the first 2 to 3 days of the

GLYCAEMIC LOAD

You may not have heard of glycaemic load, but maybe you have heard of the glycaemic index. What's the difference? The glycaemic index tells you how quickly a particular carbohydrate turns into sugar. It doesn't tell you how much of that carbohydrate is in a serving of that particular food. You need to know both things to understand a food's effect on blood sugar. That is where glycaemic load comes in. For example, the carbohydrate found in a carrot breaks down very rapidly into sugar, so it has a high glycaemic index. There isn't a lot of that carbohydrate in a serving of carrots, however, so it has a low glycaemic load. Glycaemic load gives you a better sense of how carbohydrates actually work in the diet. Here is a short list of some common foods and their glycaemic loads.

Food	Glycaemic Load	Food	Glycaemic Load
Apple	6	Jelly, sugar-free	0
Avocado	0	Lettuce (all varieties)	0
Bacon	0	Mango	8
Bagel, plain	25	Milk	4
Banana	12	Muffin	11
Beef	0	Olive oil	0
Bread, seven-grain	8	Orange	5
Bread, white	10	Pepper, sweet	0
Broccoli	0	Porridge, plain	0
Butter	0	Potato	26
Carrot	3	Raisin bran	12
Celery	0	Rice, brown	16
Cheese	0	Rice, white	14
Chicken	0	Soured cream	8
Chickpeas	8	Soya milk	8
Couscous, cooked	23	Strawberry	1
Cucumber	0	Sugar	7
Egg	0	Yoghurt, low-fat, fruit-flavoured	10
Honey	10		

diet, and each 450g (1lb) of sugar comes attached to 685g (1½lb) of water. On average, we store between 450 and 900g (1 and 2lb) of sugar in our livers. Cut out the carbs, and – poof! – 2.25kg (5lb) of sugar and water will virtually melt away.

Doctors who scoff at this say that this isn't true weight loss. You're not losing fat, just water. And the water weight will come back as soon as you reintroduce carbohydrates. Nevertheless, that early, almost effortless weight loss provides encouragement when dieters first start this eating plan, and many dieters find this useful.

A Word on Safety

Doctors have been concerned about the safety of this diet for hundreds of years. The criticism of recent generations of doctors has been that a diet so high in fat will increase your risk of heart disease by increasing cholesterol. That doesn't happen. Several recent studies have examined this issue, and it turns out that while LDL (bad) cholesterol stays about the same, HDL (good) cholesterol increases – and that reduces your risk of heart disease. And triglycerides, which increase risk of heart disease, decrease dramatically on this diet. In my own research, we looked at more than 500 diets and compared the safety and effectiveness of low-carbohydrate diets with diets that restricted fats or calories. We were particularly interested in the effects of a low-carb diet on cholesterol. We found that on average those on low-carb diets had no change in their total cholesterol. So, while many doctors remain suspicious of this diet, the research suggests that for most people this diet is safe.

THE PERFECT FIT COUNTING CARBOHYDRATES BASIC DIET

So what does the Counting Carbohydrates Diet look like? First, it is a two-part programme. In the first phase, carbohydrates are dramatically restricted. This type of limitation helps dieters lose weight immediately and continue to lose weight as long as they maintain the diet. But the sheer monotony of this diet – clearly a factor in making the diet so effective initially – also makes it virtually impossible to maintain in the long run. So, just when you are thinking that you just couldn't face another day of cheese omelettes, salmon steaks and salad, the diet adds back many of the carbohydrates you crave.

With the addition of these foods, you will be able to continue to lose weight until you reach your target. Moreover, this is a diet you will be able to continue to enjoy – a satisfying eating programme that will help you maintain your target weight, not just for now but for life.

Starting the Counting Carbohydrates Diet

In this initial phase of Counting Carbohydrates Diet, you will be restricted to a diet containing around 30 grams of carbohydrate per day. This means that the only carbohydrates you'll be able to eat are one or two servings of dairy products and green vegetables. There will be no breads, no pastries, no pastas, a very limited amount of fruits and no sweets. On the other hand, you will be able to eat your fill of seafood, meat, poultry, eggs and cheese, and many (though not all) vegetables.

Restricting your body's intake of carbohydrates to this extent will shift the way your body uses food for energy. In the diet you eat now, most of the food you take in is converted to sugar (glucose), and that sugar is the fuel used to power all the body's functions. When you start on the Counting Carbohydrates Diet and limit your carbs to 30 grams per day, you will not be eating enough sugar to run your body, so your body will switch over to its back-up fuel – fats. Your body will convert the food you eat, not to sugar, but to microscopic portions of fat, known as ketone bodies.

After several days on this diet, you'll notice many things: first, you will see an immediate change in your weight. This is the water you lose as you burn up the sugar stored in your liver. (Average weight loss will be 1.4–2.25kg/3–5lb.) You may find that you make a few extra trips to the bathroom as you lose this excess water, but that should last only a couple of days. And you may notice a slightly sweet taste in your mouth. That sweet taste is a by-product of the ketone bodies, and it proves that your body has switched over to this alternative fuel.

But I don't want you to depend on that sweet taste to tell you when your body is burning fats rather than sugar. It's not reliable enough. While you are on this initial phase of the diet, I want you to check your urine for the presence of those fat bodies. To do this you need sticks or paper strips that indicate the presence of ketones. They're available in some chemists or websites that specialize in low-carb products. When you dip the sticks or strips into your urine, they will turn pink (sometimes purple or other colours; check the label) and that will tell you if you have really got rid of enough of the carbohydrates to force your body to burn fats rather than sugar. I call this being 'in the pink'.

The main reason to check your urine daily is to make sure that you are following the diet as closely as possible. But there is an additional benefit: these ketones will help curb your appetite and that is important, especially in the early stages of a new way of eating, until you learn how to eat less and be satisfied. Portion size is, to a very large extent, learned based on portions that have satisfied you in the past. Part of any eating plan is to help you relearn a new and healthy portion size and get away from the supersize insanity that has taken hold.

In addition to checking your urine every day while on this diet, I want you to take a multivitamin every day, if you don't already. All calorie-restricted diets – not just this one – run the risk of allowing you to leave out some of the aspects of a proper diet. One vitamin a day. It's not hard, and although you may not need it, it won't hurt. I put all my patients on multivitamins. I mean, what's the downside? It doesn't really matter which multivitamin you take. Women should

GETTING 'IN THE PINK'

Sometimes it takes several days before you get 'in the pink'. If it takes longer than that, chances are you are still taking in too many carbohydrates. There are two possibilities here: first, carbohydrates are sneaking into your diet without you knowing it. This can happen very easily, so check the carbohydrate content of everything you are eating and drinking to look for hidden carbs.

Alternatively, you may be taking in only 30 grams of carbohydrate per day, but your body needs even less to make this switch. If that is the case, I would recommend eliminating all carbohydrates from your diet (including the milk in your coffee), at which point the strips will turn the proper colour; you can then add back carbs a little at a time and see at what level you start to lose that colour. That then will become your level of carbohydrate restriction.

Once you achieve this state of fat burning – once you are 'in the pink' – you need to check your urine every day to make sure you stay there. Carbohydrates are ubiquitous and it's very easy for them to find their way back onto your plate. Checking your urine every morning allows you to know that you are limiting your carbohydrates enough to lose weight. When you start to lose that colour, you need to think 'What did I eat today or yesterday that could be increasing my carbohydrate load?'

take vitamins with iron, plus calcium supplements. If you are post-menopausal, you can skip the iron – check with your doctor if you have any questions about whether you need it. For men, just the basic multivitamin should do the trick.

One last thing on this diet: make sure you drink enough water. That's eight 220ml (8fl oz) glasses per day – 1.8 litres (3 pints) of fluid – day in, day out. And coffee and alcohol don't count when you're figuring out how much you drink. One simple rule of thumb: your urine should look very much like water. If it's dark or yellow, you aren't drinking enough.

Getting enough fluid is important no matter what you are eating, but it takes on special importance with this diet. Why? Well, first of all you will be eating less of the kinds of foods that contain a lot of water. Carbohydrates contain lots of water – much more than proteins or fats. Plus, proteins in particular can increase the workload on your kidneys. You need to have enough water to flush the wastes from proteins through. Finally, ketones act as diuretics; they make you urinate more. You need to drink enough to keep up with what you put out.

I have included a list of no- and low-carbohydrate foods in this chapter as well as a 7-day eating plan for the Early Counting Carbohydrates Diet to give you some idea of how you can eat with this type of restriction. Basically, you will be eating eggs, cheese, seafood, meat and green vegetables. All are important components of the diet. Because of the nature of this diet, you will be eating a relatively high level of fat. But it will be primarily mono- and polyunsaturated fats (the 'good' fats) and relatively low in saturated fat (the bad fat).

Multiple studies have shown that, in general, low-carbohydrate dieters are able to eat this type of diet without adversely affecting their own cholesterol profile. If you are concerned about your cholesterol, however, or have a history of high LDL (bad) cholesterol, I recommend that you talk to your doctor before you start this diet and get your cholesterol rechecked after you have been on the diet for 3 to 6 months to make sure that your cholesterol is moving in the right direction.

While you can eat as much of the fats and proteins that contain no carbs as you like, everything containing carbohydrates should be measured and weighed for the first couple of weeks at least and periodically thereafter. Carbohydrates are easy to overeat and measuring them is a good reality check on what your true carbohydrate intake is.

Exactly how long you need to stay on this very restrictive phase of the diet is up to you. Between 1 and 3 months is what I generally recommend. Less than 1 month and you cheat yourself out of the benefits of this type of diet by bailing out too soon. On the other hand, most people stop losing weight (as quickly) after 3 months, usually because they can't stick to this monotonous diet any longer.

My recommendation is to follow the 30-gram Counting Carbohydrates Diet for 2 to 3 months. If you find yourself wanting to cheat (or actually cheating), then you have to consider increasing your carbohydrate content in order to give yourself some of the variety you are craving. Even though people on this diet do not value lots of variety in their diets, you are programmed at the genetic level to want some, so chances are you will. My patients certainly do.

Maintaining the Counting Carbohydrates Diet

By the time you get to this phase of the diet, you will be well on your way to your target weight. In this second phase of the Counting Carbohydrates Diet, you will be able to eat up to 100 grams of carbohydrates per day. This is still a very limited carbohydrate diet. At the most, you will be getting about a third of your calories from carbohydrates. That's about half of what the average Western diet usually provides.

But, as you probably know by now, not all carbohydrates are created equal, and so the carbohydrates you will be adding back into your diet will be limited to fruits and vegetables, with occasional whole grain pastas and breads. These carbohydrates have a low or moderate glycaemic load. You will notice that the list does not include sweets, crisps or baked goods. These high-glycaemic-index carbohydrates are foods that provide too many carbohydrates and too many calories. Moreover, because they have a moderate to high glycaemic load, they make you hungrier. These are foods that tantalize but can't satisfy. So, in this phase of the diet, the only carbohydrates allowed are complex carbs, primarily with a low glycaemic load. Fats will make up almost half of the calories consumed, and proteins fill in the rest.

On the 100-gram Counting Carbohydrates Diet, there is no need to check your urine. Once you eat this many carbohydrates, you will go back to using sugar (glucose) as your primary fuel. You will still lose weight for the same reason you were losing weight on the earlier diet: you will be eating fewer calories, and you will be avoiding the types of foods that promote high levels of insulin, since insulin can promote fat storage over fat usage.

One word of advice before you get started on this diet: the theory behind it is that by severely restricting intake of carbohydrates – the food that makes up the majority of the calories most of us take in on a given day – we will end up consuming fewer calories. The greater satisfaction associated with eating a larger percentage of your calories from proteins and fats undoubtedly contributes to this decrease in appetite. But if you end up sneaking carbohydrates back into your diet, you will be undermining the ways in which it is designed to make you lose weight. You'll end up with the worst possible diet: one that's high in fats and proteins *and* refined carbohydrates. If you add back the refined carbohydrates, you are just eating more of everything, and that is a sure way to gain weight.

On the other hand, if you feel good on this diet, and if it allows you to achieve and maintain your desired weight, there is no reason to stop it once you have achieved your ideal weight. This diet is balanced enough to allow you to continue on it indefinitely.

Now, on to the foods and the diet!

FOOD LIST FOR THE COUNTING CARBS BASIC DIET

NO CARBOHYDRATE CONTENT

MEAT, POULTRY AND SEAFOOD (Virtually all are carbohydrate-free – exceptions found in Very Low Carb Foods list on the next page.)

FATS AND OILS

Almond oil

Avocado oil

Margarine

Olive oil

Rapeseed oil

Sesame oil

Shortening

Soya bean oil

Sunflower oil

VEGETABLES

Lettuce

Rocket

Watercress

CHEESE AND OTHER DAIRY PRODUCTS

Babybel

Blue cheese

Brie

Butter

Camembert

Emmenthal

Fontina cheese

Havarti cheese

SPICES AND CONDIMENTS

Capers

Lemon juice

Mayonnaise

Mustard

Sugar substitutes

Vinegar

BEVERAGES

Coffee

Soft drinks, diet

Clear soup, beef and chicken stock

Tea

Water (including unsweetened flavoured varieties and carbonated)

SWEETS

Jelly (sugar-free)

VERY LOW CARB FOODS (This list provides you with the serving sizes that will give you around 5 grams of carbohydrates; these aren't the amounts you must eat, but they will give you an idea of how much carbohydrate is contained in these naturally low-carb foods.)

MEAT, POULTRY AND SEAFOOD

Abalone	90g/3oz
Caviar	145g/5oz
Clams	90g/3oz/5 clams
Eggs	5 eggs
Frankfurters	5 franks
Ham	285g/10oz
Lobster	170g/6oz
Luncheon meats	2 slices
Mussels	90g/3oz
Oysters	90g/3oz/6 cooked
Pâté	115g/4oz
Roe	170g/6oz
Sausage	145g/5oz
Scallops	170g/6oz/10 pieces
Squid, fried	90g/3oz

NUTS AND SEEDS

Almond butter	2 tbsp
Almonds	30g/1oz
Brazil nuts	6–8 nuts
Cashews	30g/1oz
Hazelnuts	30g/1oz
Macadamia nuts	45g/1½oz
Peanut butter	2 tbsp
Peanuts	30g/1oz

Pecans	20 halves
Pine nuts	45g/1½oz
Pistachio nuts	30g/1oz
Sunflower seeds	20g/¾oz
Walnuts	30g/1oz

FRUITS AND VEGETABLES

Apricot	1 medium fruit
Artichoke hearts	90g/3oz/4 pieces
Asparagus	10 medium spears
Aubergine	200g/7oz
Avocado	1 medium
Bamboo shoots	75g/2½oz
Blueberries, fresh	25 berries
Beans, green	145g/5oz
Beans, mung, cooked	30g/1oz
Beans, runner	200g/7oz
Bean sprouts	145g/5oz
Broccoli florets	200g/7oz
Cabbage, savoy	75g/2½oz
Cauliflower	200g/7oz
Celeriac	100g/3½oz
Celery	5 large sticks
Coleslaw	100g/3½oz
Courgettes	275g/9¼oz
Cucumber	145g/5oz
Endive, raw	145g/5oz
Gherkins	145g/5oz
Kale	100g/3½oz
Mangetout	15 pods
Mushrooms	145g/5oz
Okra	30 pods
Olives	15
Peppers, green	1 medium

FRUITS AND VEGETABLES (CONT.)

Pickles, sweet	30g/1oz
Radishes	225g/8oz
Raspberries, fresh	25 berries
Shallots	30g/1oz
Spinach	375g/13oz
Spring onions	115g/4oz
Squash, butternut	75g/2½oz
Strawberries	90g/3oz
Swiss chard	150g/5½oz
Tomato, canned	170g/6oz
Tomato, fresh	1 whole
Turnip, cooked	250g/9oz

DAIRY

Anchor Light aerosol cream	5 tbsp
Cream, single	120ml/4fl oz
Milk, whole or semi-skimmed	120ml/4fl oz
Soured cream	120ml/4fl oz
Yoghurt, plain	80ml/3fl oz
Yoghurt, drinking	50ml/3 tbsp

CHEESE

Note: the amount of carbohydrate in cheeses varies across brands. Therefore the amount listed here represents the very highest carb content you are likely to find.

Bel paese	145g/5oz
Cheddar	145g/5oz
Cottage cheese	90g/3oz
Cream cheese	170g/6oz
Edam	145g/5oz
Feta	145g/5oz
Gouda	145g/5oz
Jarlsberg	145g/5oz

Lancashire	145g/5oz
Leicester	145g/5oz
Mozzarella	145g/5oz
Parmesan	145g/5oz
Processed	145g/5oz/5 slices
Processed, low-fat	145g/5oz/5 slices
Provolone	145g/5oz
Ricotta	145g/5oz
Romano	145g/5oz
String cheese	145g/5oz

CONDIMENTS

Gravy (most canned and mix varieties)	60ml/2fl oz
Horseradish	115g/4oz
Jam	1 tsp
Ketchup	1 tbsp
Miso	2 tbsp
Salad dressing (except low-fat)	2 tbsp
Salsa	145g/5oz
Sauces (most – some big exceptions, so check label)	2 tbsp
Sesame butter (tahini)	2 tbsp
Soup, onion	240ml/8fl oz
Tofu, silken	170g/6oz

DAILY MEAL PLANS
FOR THE 30-GRAM COUNTING CARBS DIET

(Dishes in **bold print** are listed alphabetically in the recipe section at the end of the chapter, on page 148.)

DAY

Breakfast

3-egg omelette (use only 1–2 yolks but all 3 whites) with ham and 60g (2oz) low-fat Cheddar cheese (cook in olive oil)	3.5g
Coffee with semi-skimmed milk and sweetener (not sugar)	1.5g

AM Snack

90g (3oz) cottage cheese with 60g (2oz) cucumbers and 2–3 radishes	5.5g

Lunch

Chef salad made with ½ head of lettuce and 75g (2½oz) spinach, 30g (1oz) low-fat cheese, ham, 1 hard-boiled egg, and 4 artichoke hearts dressed with **Vinaigrette** (if you use bottled salad dressing, check the carb content – should be 0)	4g

PM Snack

½ avocado with **Vinaigrette**	3g

Dinner

Chicken breast dredged in Parmesan cheese and sautéed in olive oil	0g

Broccoli florets with lemon juice	3g
10 spears asparagus	4g
75g (2½oz) raw spinach salad and 2–3 hearts of palm	4g
Total carbohydrates	**28.5g**

DAY

Breakfast

60g (2oz) smoked salmon and cream cheese	1g
1 tomato, sliced	6g
Coffee with semi-skimmed milk and sweetener	1.5g

AM Snack

Celery spread with 2 tablespoons cream cheese	2g

Lunch

Cold Tomato Stuffed with Seafood (try adding capers for a more sophisticated taste)	6g

PM Snack

3 ham and low-fat cheese rolls (1 slice low-fat ham, 1 slice low-fat Gruyère or Emmenthal, with a dab of mustard, rolled up)	2g

Dinner

115g (4oz) grilled swordfish	0g
45g (1½oz) sautéed mushrooms	5g
100g (3½oz) rocket and lettuce salad with cucumbers and radishes topped with **Vinaigrette**	1g
Sugar-free jelly with 2 tablespoons Anchor Light aerosol cream	2g
Total carbohydrates	**26.5g**

DAY

Breakfast

Scrambled eggs (use 2 egg whites and 1 egg yolk)	1.5g
2 slices back bacon	0g
Coffee with semi-skimmed milk and sweetener	1.5g

AM Snack

10–12 macadamia nuts	4g

Lunch

Caesar salad (romaine lettuce, slivers of Parmesan cheese, no croutons, in Caesar dressing – check label for carb content) topped with 90g (3oz) grilled chicken breast	4g

PM Snack

Celery spread with 30g (1oz) cream cheese	1g

Dinner

Grilled lamb chop, served with sautéed mushrooms and onions	5g
10 asparagus spears, steamed	5g
Broccoli florets, steamed	3g
Total carbohydrates	**25g**

DAY

Breakfast

120ml (4fl oz) low-fat natural yoghurt	8g
90g (3oz) sliced strawberries	5g
2 slices back bacon	0g
Coffee with semi-skimmed milk and sweetener	1.5g

AM Snack

30g (1oz) salmon spread with 2 tablespoons cream cheese	1g

Lunch

Cold Tomato Stuffed with Seafood	6g
240ml (8fl oz) low-fat chicken consommé	0g
5 green olives	1g

PM Snack

3 ham and low-fat cheese rolls	2g

Dinner

Filet mignon, grilled	0g
Lettuce and tomato salad (½ head lettuce and 1–2 tomatoes)	5g
Asparagus or Green Beans Parmesan	5g
Total carbohydrates	**34.5g**

DAY 5

Breakfast

Mushroom omelette made with 3 egg whites and 1 or 2 egg yolks and 60g (2oz) sautéed mushrooms	5.5g
2 slices back bacon	0g
Coffee with semi-skimmed milk and sweetener	1.5g

AM Snack

15 olives	5g

Lunch

240ml (8fl oz) onion soup	5g
115g (4oz) prawn salad (boiled prawns, celery, onion, and 2 tablespoons mayonnaise) served on bed of greens and radicchio	5g

PM Snack

Celery spread with 30g (1oz) cream cheese   1g

Dinner

Chicken Mediterranean   4g

Lettuce and tomato salad (made with
½ head lettuce and 1 tomato) with
Creamy Vinaigrette   5g

Total carbohydrates   **32g**

DAY

Breakfast

2 poached eggs on back bacon served on a bed
of steamed spinach (75g/3½oz raw) with 2 tablespoons
Hollandaise Sauce, if desired   3g

Coffee with semi-skimmed milk and sweetener   1.5g

AM Snack

47 pistachio nuts   5g

Lunch

Spinach salad with bacon, 1 hard-boiled egg,
and 30g (1oz) walnuts with **Vinaigrette** or other
no-carb dressing   6g

PM Snack

60g (2oz) cheese   2g

Dinner

Grilled king prawns   1g

100g (3½oz) endive salad with no-carb dressing   2g

Spaghetti squash, steamed, served with butter and
Parmesan cheese   5g

Sugar-free jelly with 2 tablespoons Anchor Light
aerosol cream   2g

Total carbohydrates   **27.5g**

DAY

Breakfast

2 poached eggs	1g
2 slices back bacon	0g
½ tomato, sliced, grilled if desired	3g
Coffee with semi-skimmed milk and sweetener	1.5g

AM Snack

240ml (8fl oz) onion soup	5g
30g (1oz) blueberries	5g

Lunch

115g (4oz) grilled chicken (skinless)	0g
Cucumber, onion and watercress salad with **Vinaigrette** or other no-carb dressing	5g

PM Snack

Roast beef, sliced and rolled	0g

Dinner

Tuna steak, grilled, dressed with 60ml (2fl oz) salsa	2g
100g (3½oz) **Coleslaw**	6g
Broccoli florets, steamed, with ½ teaspoon butter and squeeze of lemon juice	2g
Total carbohydrates	**30.5g**

RECIPES FOR CARBOHYDRATE COUNTERS

※

For your convenience, the recipes are listed in alphabetical order.

ASPARAGUS OR GREEN BEANS PARMESAN

450–900g (1–2lb) asparagus or 300g (10½oz) whole green
   beans, topped and tailed
15–30g (½–1oz) butter
Salt
Ground black pepper
60g (2oz) thinly sliced fresh Parmesan

Place a steamer basket in a large pot with 2.5cm (1in) of water. Bring to the boil over a high heat. Place the asparagus or green beans in the basket, reduce the heat to medium and steam until almost ready to eat, about 8 to 10 minutes. Rinse with cold water to prevent further cooking. Place in a buttered casserole dish. Dot with butter and add salt and pepper to taste. Top with 45g (1½oz) of the cheese. Bake at 230°C (450°F) gas 8 until the cheese is just beginning to turn brown. Remove from the oven, sprinkle with the remaining Parmesan, and serve.

MAKES 4 SERVINGS
PER SERVING: 5G CARBOHYDRATES

CHICKEN MEDITERRANEAN

4 tablespoons olive oil
4 chicken legs

1 onion, sliced

1 can (400g/14oz) whole tomatoes

240ml (8fl oz) white wine

1 clove garlic, crushed

Salt

Ground black pepper

Black olives (optional)

Heat the oil in a large saucepan over a medium-high heat. Add the chicken and cook until browned. Remove from the saucepan. Add the onion to the same pan and cook until transparent but not brown. Add the tomatoes, wine and garlic. Add salt and pepper to taste. Add the olives, if using. Replace the chicken in the saucepan. Cover, reduce heat to low, and cook for 20 minutes, or until the chicken is cooked through.

MAKES 4 SERVINGS
PER SERVING: 4G CARBOHYDRATES

COLD TOMATOES STUFFED WITH SEAFOOD

4 firm unpeeled tomatoes

Salt

STUFFING

1 can (170g/6oz) tuna or crab

1 onion, chopped

1–2 sticks celery, chopped

1 green pepper, chopped

Salt

Ground black pepper

3 tablespoons mayonnaise

Lettuce

Vinaigrette (page 152)

Cut a cavity in the stem end of each of the tomatoes, sprinkle with salt, and invert on a rack to drain as you prepare the stuffing.

To make the stuffing: In a bowl, mix together the tuna or crab, with the onion, celery and pepper. Add salt and black pepper to taste. Add the mayonnaise (the mixture should be wet but not gooey).

Fill the tomatoes with the seafood salad and serve on a bed of lettuce lightly dressed with Vinaigrette.

MAKES 4 SERVINGS
PER SERVING: 6G CARBOHYDRATES

COLESLAW

1 small head cabbage, thinly sliced
3 sticks celery, thinly sliced
2–3 spring onions, thinly sliced
1 green pepper, finely diced
1 small apple, peeled, cored and finely sliced
1 medium cucumber, peeled, seeded and thinly sliced
120ml (4fl oz) mayonnaise
80ml (3fl oz) soured cream
½ tablespoon Dijon mustard
2 tablespoons wine vinegar or cider vinegar
1 teaspoon salt
¼ teaspoon caraway seeds
¼ teaspoon celery seeds
Ground black pepper

In a large bowl, combine the cabbage, celery, spring onions, pepper, apple and cucumber. In a small bowl, mix the mayonnaise, soured cream, mustard, vinegar, salt, caraway seeds and celery seeds. Mix into the cabbage mixture and add black pepper to taste.

MAKES 10 SERVINGS
PER SERVING: 6G CARBOHYDRATES

CREAMY VINAIGRETTE

1 egg
60ml (2fl oz) good quality vinegar
1 teaspoon Dijon mustard
1 teaspoon shallots, finely chopped
180ml (6fl oz) olive oil
Salt
Ground black pepper

In a blender, combine the egg, vinegar, mustard and shallots. Blend until smooth. With the blender running at a low speed, drizzle in the oil. When the mixture is creamy and quite thick, add salt and pepper to taste. The mixture will thicken in the refrigerator. Add 1 to 2 teaspoons warm water to achieve the consistency you like.

MAKES 12 SERVINGS
PER SERVING: 1G CARBOHYDRATES

HOLLANDAISE SAUCE

115g (4oz) butter
3 egg yolks
½ teaspoon salt
1 tablespoon lemon juice
Pinch of mustard powder

Melt the butter in a saucepan over a low heat, making sure it doesn't burn. In a blender, combine the egg yolks, salt, lemon juice and mustard powder. With the blender running, drizzle in the melted butter. The mixture will thicken. Add more lemon juice or seasoning if desired. Use immediately or keep warm by putting in a bowl and nesting the bowl in another bowl filled with very hot water. It will keep for up to 30 minutes this way.

MAKES 6 SERVINGS
PER SERVING: 0G CARBOHYDRATES

VINAIGRETTE

50ml (1½fl oz) olive oil
50ml (1½fl oz) wine vinegar
50ml (1½fl oz) water
1–2 cloves garlic, crushed
Salt
Ground black pepper

In a small bowl, mix together the oil, vinegar, water and garlic. Add salt and pepper to taste.

MAKES 6 SERVINGS
PER SERVING: 1G CARBOHYDRATES

❋ *You can replace up to half of the vinegar with mustard –*
  Dijon mustard works best.

CHAPTER 7

THE COUNTING CALORIES DIET

ALTHOUGH YOU WON'T KNOW MY PATIENT JANET, YOU'VE PROBABLY known someone like her. Or maybe you are that someone.

Janet is 32. She works in a high-powered law firm in Washington, DC. She's divorced, with two children. Janet was pretty active as a kid and teenager. She loved sports, especially swimming and tennis. She was never skinny; she had broad shoulders and some real muscle. Although she was big, she never thought of herself as fat. After college came working 9 to 5, then marriage and two children. Suddenly, by her mid-twenties, Janet found herself overweight. She wanted to lose weight, but she didn't really know how. She tried diets – lots of diets.

Janet's best success had come with a low-carbohydrate, high-protein diet. As a teenager she had lost weight with the Scarsdale diet.

Then she'd tried the Atkins diet, the Protein Power diet, the Carbo-hydrate Addict's diet. They all worked for a while, but eventually she found herself gorging on bread and potatoes. She told me that at one point she felt as if she would kill for corn on the cob. She never felt hungry, it's true. But she never felt satisfied either. And without sat-isfaction, she couldn't stick to the diet, and she would revert to her old ways of eating.

The last few years she'd been trying the low-fat diets. They sounded healthier and allowed her the carbs she so loved. 'I've Pri-tikined, I've tried to Stop the Madness, but I couldn't. It just didn't work.' On these diets, mealtime seemed to mean huge and depressing piles of salad or vegetables. And although she did get to eat the pasta and bread she wanted, she'd felt hungry, tired and really, really cranky.

She came to me, she said, because she couldn't afford another 'success' like she'd had in the past. 'Another diet that ends up putting 20 pounds on me, and I just don't know what I'd do.'

The traditional view of weight loss is that it's really just a little maths problem: 'Oh, if I eat 500 fewer calories, I'll lose that much in weight. Great.' You wouldn't be reading this book if it were that easy.

It is true that reducing the number of calories you consume is an essential component of losing weight, and what *all* diets do is arrange what you eat so that you do, in fact, take in fewer calories. The trick to any successful diet is to eat fewer calories but to do it in a way that fools your body and brain into feeling that you are satisfied and never hungry. Low-fat diets try to do this by giving you unlimited amounts of fruits and vegetables and helping you fill up on real stick-to-the-ribs foods like pasta, grains and starchy beans. Low-carb diets try to bore you to thinness by giving you access to all the meat you can eat, and betting that the satisfying aspect of meats and proteins and the monotony of the diet will help you to simply eat less of these high-calorie foods.

A diet that counts calories gets rid of these somewhat arbitrary limits on foods and allows you to eat all types of food. The trick in this diet – since they all have one – is to direct you to the foods that are the most satisfying and most filling in all food categories. By doing this, we can use the foods that work well in the low-fat diets and the low-carb diets, and we can satisfy one of the most basic needs we all have – the real need for variety in the foods we eat. A diet that explicitly tries to reduce calories can help many people lose weight. If you have filled out the questionnaire and arrived at this chapter, it is because you are one of those people.

In this chapter, we will look at who does well on a calorie-counting diet and which diet characteristics can make this way of eating successful. I have also provided a list of low-calorie foods and a 7-day eating plan. Finally, I've given you some simple recipes that can help you incorporate many of these principles into meals you can enjoy for a lifetime.

Who are the people who do well on, and what makes them compatible with, a low-calorie diet? First and foremost, these are individuals who need variety in their diets. Not everyone does. Some people eat the same thing for dinner 3 or 4 days a week and enjoy that. You are not one of those people. You crave variety in taste, in texture, in aroma, in richness. You've fallen off the diet wagon because of boredom and impatience with the unending sameness of the foods available to you.

In fact, monotony is one of the weight-loss tools used in many diets, though they probably won't tell you that. The same-old–same-old dampens appetite, at least for a time. Eventually, though, most of us crave variety at some level. It is hardwired into us as a mechanism to ensure we get the full range of nutrients we need. For those people who do well on a diet that looks only at calorie content, the variety and sensory qualities of foods are vital in order for them to feel satisfied.

Do you find yourself at the end of the day standing in front of the refrigerator with the door open, looking for something crunchy or sour or aromatic or rich after the bland nourishments of a low-fat diet with all its veggies and pasta? Or do you crave the refreshing crispness of a partially ripe pear after a few days of steak and more steak on a low-carbohydrate diet? Then welcome to the Counting Calories Diet. This is where you belong.

TESSA'S STORY

I first met Tessa just after her husband had his second heart attack. He was going to be okay, but his illness made her aware of her own risks. At 68, she was still energetic and had a lively disposition. She'd retired from her banking job a few years earlier and these days devoted her time to volunteer work and her grandchildren. When she walked into my office, she moved with energy and a briskness that made her appear much younger than the age on her driver's licence. She was pretty healthy: she had high blood pressure that was well-controlled on one medicine, and her LDL (bad) cholesterol was a little too high, though she wasn't taking any medicine for it. She used to exercise regularly but had got out of the habit these past few years, and now her knees bothered her when she walked too far.

Her weight had been up and down most of her adult life, though, she said quickly, she'd never been this heavy before. When she was younger, she could lose weight just by watching what she ate, but that hadn't worked for quite a while. A few years ago she'd had some success with Weight Watchers but found the regular meetings burdensome. She'd also had some success with ready-prepared diet meals, but she loved to cook so this strategy was short lived. She'd never tried a low-carbohydrate diet – although she'd bought the books. She couldn't imagine limiting herself to the few foods allowed on that diet. She kept a diet diary and filled out the questionnaire.

Tessa, like Janet, is a classic calorie-counting dieter.

Why? First of all, they both craved variety in their diets. Tessa knew that about herself. Janet had to find out the hard way – through trial and failure. It was clear from their diet diaries and their diet histories that they craved variety in taste, texture, aroma and richness. Janet had fallen off the diet wagon because of boredom with the unending sameness of the foods available to her. Tessa wouldn't even try those types of diets. Variety was the key to their satisfaction, and only a low-calorie diet will allow them to choose from the full palette of foods.

Another important quality in these dieters was the recognition that more food was not what they wanted; what they craved was more kinds of foods. That is the essential trade-off in a low-calorie diet and is at the heart of its success. In a low-fat diet, you trade eating a high-calorie, high-fat food for the pleasure of eating more of a low-fat, low-calorie food. In a low-carb diet, you trade the volume of a high-carbohydrate diet for one rich in fats and proteins. In the low-calorie diet, you trade eating a lot of any single food for a chance to eat a little of a lot of different foods. This was a bargain Tessa and Janet were willing to make. Tessa recognized that controlling portions was central to the success of diets she'd tried in the past. And she knew she'd never felt hungry on smaller portions. Janet came to this from the other direction. She'd tried the all-you-can-eat-of-one-food diets and had come away wanting different food – not more food.

THE BASICS
OF A CALORIE-COUNTING DIET

You don't hear many people raving about their wildly successful calorie-counting diets these days. That's because if you cut calories willy-nilly, if you cut high-calorie foods and try to live only on low-calorie foods without choosing the foods that will help keep you feeling full, you will be hungry and will fail. This is the diet of iceberg lettuce with low-fat dressing. This is the diet of tuna and melba toast. They lack variety; they lack substance; they leave you hungry; they doom you to failure. A basic principle in dieting is that you must eat foods that you like and eat in a way that satisfies you, or you won't be able to stay on the diet. It's a law of nature almost as immutable as gravity.

Recently, a couple of cereal companies recommended a low-calorie diet that featured their cereals prominently (naturally). The idea was to eat this diet cereal for breakfast and for lunch and then eat a normal dinner. Liquid diet products also advocated this type of calorie-restricted diet. Drink a can of diet meal replacement for breakfast and lunch and then eat a modest-size dinner at night. Here's the problem: there is no way that by the end of the day you are going to be able to eat a modest-size dinner. By the time you sit down to dinner, you are starving! And, if you are someone who craves variety, you haven't got any by the time you reach dinner.

These diets sell themselves as reasonable alternatives, but in fact they are virtually impossible to follow. And when you fail on them, do you blame the company for suggesting an unreasonable way to lose weight? No, chances are you do not. Chances are you condemn yourself for a lack of willpower. I'm here to tell you that no one can stand up to real hunger. It goes against the way our bodies are put together. To succeed, you must choose foods that maximize your sense of fullness and satisfy the parts of you that need to be satisfied.

How can you do that?

First, on a low-calorie diet – or on any diet for that matter – you need to focus on foods that make you feel full and keep you feeling full until it's time for you to eat again. Each of the three food components – carbs, fats and proteins – has an important role in making you feel full. Carbohydrates, especially those high in fibre and low on the glycaemic load, provide bulk or volume. High-fibre carbs also stay in your stomach longer, which also promotes a feeling of long-lasting fullness. Proteins, and to a lesser extent fat, provide a sense of satiety by triggering a variety of digestive enzymes. Many of these enzymes have the job of communicating to your brain that you have eaten.

Proteins are the most filling food type – they play a role in making you feel full, and there is good evidence that they also play an important role in helping to prolong that feeling of fullness. Next are complex (that is, low-glycaemic-load) carbohydrates, then last but not least, come fats, which don't seem to contribute to an immediate sense of fullness but make you feel full for longer.

Thus, each meal should be made up of proteins, complex carbohydrates and some fat. The real bonus of a calorie-counting diet is that you can eat all three types of foods based on what works best for you. The ideal proportion of these depends on the individual. You need to figure out what makes you full, but on a low-calorie diet I recommend eating a big portion of low-glycaemic-load, high-fibre, unrefined carbohydrates (between 45 and 50 per cent of the calories in a meal), and splitting the remainder between proteins (15 to 25 per cent) and fats (35 to 40 per cent).

Here's another important point to remember while following a calorie-counting diet: you must eat when you are hungry, not when you are starving. If you allow yourself to get really, really hungry, it becomes very difficult to make yourself stop once you finally get a chance to eat. This is true no matter what diet you are following, but it takes on particular importance in a calorie-counting diet, because portion control is such an important aspect of the diet.

Moreover, when you are really hungry, it is virtually impossible to resist any temptation. If you walk by a bowl of chocolates or crisps when you are starving, the chance that you will be able to just walk on by drops dramatically. Your ability to pass McDonald's or the bakery on your way home is also impaired. You might be able to do it much of the time – though it's hard work – but you won't be able to do it all of the time. So plan to have three meals a day as well as one or two snacks. This way, you will increase your chances of eating what you should eat and responding to the body's cues when you have eaten enough.

A third strategy for a successful calorie-counting diet: try to eat most of your calories early in the day. Breakfast should contain around one-third of the calories you are planning to eat that day. This is a more natural way to eat – providing your body with the fuel it needs to take on the day – and it maximizes your body's ability to burn the calories you take in over the course of the day. It also sends you into the evening with less hunger, and that's important, because the social aspect of dinner makes it an ideal opportunity to overeat. It's a lot easier to pass up that opportunity if you are hungry but not starving when dinnertime comes around.

Try to eat a variety of foods, tastes and textures at every meal since, if you are reading this chapter, chances are that variety is an important signal of satisfaction. Maximize the satiety signals you send your body by eating the variety you crave.

PORTION: THE KEY TO SUCCESS

The final aspect of a low-calorie diet that needs to be discussed is portion size. Thanks to the supersize world we live in, our sense of portion size is way out of control. When you start eating huge portions that have too many calories, you're likely to feel uncomfortable at first, even sick. But after a surprisingly short time, you get used to that portion size, and if you get less, you feel that the smaller portion is too small. Your eyes get used to seeing a certain amount of food on the plate as a visual cue to how much is enough. Your eyes become accustomed to different portion sizes quickly – much more quickly than your stomach – and you learn to eat bigger (or, more rarely, smaller) portions quite easily.

But this is the world we find ourselves in: we crave variety and voilà! – it's there, 24/7. We crave big steaming portions that fill up bigger and bigger plates. We get that too. And we have foods that are targeted to our most primaeval needs: lots of fat, lots of carbs. That is a diet for widespread obesity. The United Kingdom is on such a diet. And it's working.

Our job is to figure out a way to eat in this world so that our bodies look and act the way we want them to, not the way fast-food corporations want them to. That's what this book is all about. We live in a culture where we can eat pretty much anything we want, whenever we want and as much as we want. It's up to us to decide how to eat.

So, does a low-calorie diet work? Just ask Tessa. She'd lost 16kg (35lb) 6 months after starting this diet, and she's still going strong. And Janet has neared her target size. She's actually had to buy a whole new wardrobe. It worked for them; it could work for you too.

THE PERFECT FIT COUNTING CALORIES BASIC DIET

Enough about principle; on to practice.

In a diet that focuses on counting calories, there are really only two questions: how many and what. Specifically, how many calories should you eat per day and what foods will make up those calories.

Let's start with how many. I recommend that most people start with a 1,200-calorie diet. Before you roll your eyes and grab your stomach, let me tell you why. Our bodies are designed to love staying the same. We hate change at the most basic level. You can see this with weight gain – even though we are purposefully designed to gain weight more easily than we lose weight. Most people have to overeat for several days (and for some lucky few, even weeks) before they see a change in the way their clothes fit or notice a change on the scales. Our bodies seek stability; if the body can avoid change, it does. Research has shown us over and over again that you can increase the number of calories in a person's diet, and he or she will maintain the same weight – although not for too long.

It's the same thing with weight loss. If you reduce your calories by 500 calories a day (basically, one bagel or two colas less per day), then theoretically you would lose 450g (1lb) in 7 days. That's the theory; the reality is that because our bodies resist change, you don't lose that weight. Physics says you will; our bodies give a raspberry to physics, at least for a while. We resist weight gain by increasing (ever so slightly) our metabolism. We resist weight loss by decreasing (again, ever so slightly) our metabolism. Moreover, if you eliminate those calories while maintaining the same essential diet – except for the foods you are cutting out – you will probably get hungry, and you may not be able to consistently get rid of those 500 calories. So if you cut back your diet by 500 calories, you will lose weight, but it may take a while for that change to make itself known on the scales or in your clothes.

To get around this little obstacle, I put most of my patients on a 1,200-calorie diet to get things jump-started. At 1,200 calories, you probably will see a 450- to 900-g (1- to 2-lb) weight change per week, and chances are, if you follow the diet and eat foods that will fill your stomach and satisfy your need for variety, you will be able to eat those paltry (you think) 1,200 calories and not get hungry.

Who shouldn't be on a 1,200-calorie-a-day diet? If you really stick to the diet and find that you are hungry, then you should consider increasing your daily calorie intake to 1,500 calories a day. Most of my patients do well on a 1,200-calorie-a-day diet. A few, mostly men, have needed 1,500 calories a day; a couple who were very overweight have needed 1,800 calories. But in general, most can tolerate this level of calorie reduction pretty well.

I recommend that you try the 1,200 calories for 4 to 5 days. Make sure you are eating three meals a day; make sure you are snacking; make sure you are eating foods from each of the three food types (proteins, carbohydrates and fats). And if you find that you are still unsatisfied, up the calorie content by 300 calories. If you still feel hungry, up it again. You won't be able to follow a diet if you are hungry, so increase the calorie content until you are comfortable and feel satisfied but not overly full at the end of each meal. Another tip, if you are not hungry for your next snack or meal, then you probably ate too much at your last meal. When that happens, reduce your portion even more.

Now, what should you be eating? Lots of carbohydrates, certainly. These should be high-fibre, low-glycaemic-load carbs. What that really means is that you will be eating plenty of fruits and vegetables, some whole grain bread and some pastas and rice. You will see from the 7-day eating plan that almost half of your calories will come from foods like this. You will be eating lots of dairy products – the low-fat variety, since the fat in most dairy products is saturated and promotes heart disease in many people. You will be eating meat, poultry or fish every day. Again, I encourage you to choose the low-fat versions of these foods, because the fats contained in them are primarily saturated fats. You won't be avoiding fat – up to 40 per cent of your calories will come from fat – but it will be primarily mono- and polyunsaturated fat (from olive oil and nuts) and omega fats (from fish).

To make this work, it's important to keep a food diary. Write down everything you eat and drink. I think I've convinced you that it's hard to know what you eat unless you write it down. Now that you are changing the way you eat, it's more important than ever. I also recommend that you measure everything you eat, at least initially. You might think you know how much you are eating, but I bet if you measured it out you would be surprised. You will learn pretty quickly how much meat makes up a 115-g (4-oz) serving, so you won't have to do this forever. But you should weigh and measure everything for the first 2 weeks of this eating plan.

You will notice that I have not included very many ready-prepared foods. That's because most of those foods include fats and sugars as preservatives. These are empty calories. Some people call sweets empty calories because they provide sugar without any other nutrients. I think there is a place for sweets in a balanced diet. But calories that are added just to make the food last longer on the shelf or in the freezer are truly empty calories. They work for the manufacturer, but not for you. Moreover, many processed foods – particularly baked goods like breads, pastries and muffins – contain trans fats. Trans fats promote heart disease and are found in only tiny amounts in unprocessed foods. Manufacturers developed these fats to replace butter but did too good a job. It turns out that they act very much like butter in your system, so just leave them out of your diet. (If you want to know more about saturated fat, like butter, and trans fats, see chapter 9.)

On this low-calorie diet, you should lose 450 to 900g (1 to 2lb) per week. If after 2 weeks you haven't lost weight, check your diary to see what you have been eating. Have you eaten other foods? Which other foods? Why did you eat them? Is there any way to fit them in without blowing your calorie limit? Consider the possibility that 1,200 calories are too many for you. I have several patients who needed to reduce their intake to 1,000 calories per day. This is a science experiment, and you are the test tube. No one can tell you exactly what to eat to make yourself feel good and weigh the right amount. In the final analysis, you have to figure out what makes you feel good and how to eat that way.

On the following pages I've listed some foods, but I've listed them in amounts that will give you 100 calories. That could be 1½ medium-size artichokes or four crackers. I've listed them in categories: protein, carbs and fats. You need to eat some from each column in order to maximize your feeling of fullness. So nearly half of your calories will come from carbohydrates (fruits, vegetables, starches), up to 20 per cent of your calories will come from proteins (meats, poultry, seafood, dairy products and nuts) and 35 to 40 per cent of your calories will come from fats.

I've also provided a 7-day eating plan to let you see how you might put all this together, and I end this chapter with a few recipes that have been helpful to my patients and to me. In fact, Tessa and Janet both have given me recipes that they have found helpful in their new way of eating.

SIX TIPS FOR CALORIE COUNTERS

1. Eat foods that make you feel full: carbs that contain fibre and have a low glycaemic load; low-fat (lower-calorie) proteins; and some amount of fat. You must eat all three in each meal or snack.

2. Eat when you are hungry, not when you are starving.

3. Get your calories in early – breakfast is a must; try to have at least two-thirds of your calories before dinner.

4. Variety can mean more work, but it's a powerful satisfier. Don't skimp on sources of satisfaction.

5. Portion size is key; measure your portions until you know what you are eating.

6. Keep a diet diary – knowledge is power.

FOOD LIST FOR THE COUNTING CALORIES BASIC DIET

PROTEINS	100-CALORIE PORTION

MEAT, POULTRY AND SEAFOOD (115g/4oz is considered a normal serving size, and this assumes that meats are cooked without adding fats.)

Beef

Rump steak, lean only	45g/1½oz
Silverside (pot roast)	45g/1½oz
Topside, roasted	60g/2oz

Pork

Bacon (streaky)	2 slices
Back bacon	75g/2½oz
Ham	45g/1½oz
Pork chop	60g/2oz

Poultry

Chicken, no skin	60g/2oz
Chicken, with skin	45g/1½oz
Turkey, no skin	90g/3oz
Turkey, with skin	60g/2oz

Seafood

Clams	115g/4oz/8 clams
Flounder	90g/3oz
Oysters	90g/3oz/10 oysters
Prawns	115g/4oz/15 prawns
Salmon, fresh	60g/2oz
Salmon, smoked	90g/3oz
Tuna, fresh	75g/2½oz
Tuna, brine-packed	60g/2oz

CHEESE

Brie	30g/1oz
Cheddar, low-fat	60g/2oz

Feta	45g/1½oz
Gruyère or Emmenthal	30g/1oz
Mozzarella	30g/1oz
Mozzarella, low-fat	45g/1½oz
Parmesan	30g/1oz
Processed	30g/1oz/1 slice
Processed, low-fat	60g/2oz/2 slices
String cheese	30g/1oz

DAIRY

Eggs	1 large
Milk, skimmed	350ml/12fl oz
Milk, semi-skimmed	200ml/7fl oz
Milk, whole	150ml/5fl oz

NUTS

Almonds	15g/½oz
Cashews	15g/½oz
Peanuts, roasted	15g/½oz
Pecans	15g/½oz
Pistachio nuts	15g/½oz

CARBOHYDRATES	100-CALORIE PORTION

VEGETABLES

Asparagus, canned	400g/14oz
Asparagus, fresh	25 spears
Artichoke, fresh	1½ medium globes
Aubergine, peeled	1 medium
Avocado, fresh	⅓ medium
Beans, green, fresh	400g/14oz
Beans, kidney, cooked	100g/3½oz
Beans, butter	125g/4½oz
Beetroot	20 slices
Black-eyed peas	100g/3½oz

CARBOHYDRATES	100-CALORIE PORTION
VEGETABLES (CONT.)	
Broccoli	400g/14oz
Brussels sprouts	400g/14oz
Cabbage	½ head
Carrots, fresh	5 large whole
Cauliflower	½ head
Celery	10 whole sticks
Courgettes	700g/1lb 9oz
Cucumber	2½ whole
Lentils, cooked	100g/3½oz
Lettuce	1 large head
Peas, cooked	200g/7oz
Peas, raw	170g/6oz
Sugar snap peas	170g/6oz
Peppers	4 whole
Potato, baked	½ medium
Potato, sweet	1 medium
Spinach	500g/1lb 2oz
Squash, acorn, cooked	170g/6oz
Sweetcorn	90g/3oz
Tomato, canned	5 medium
Tomato, fresh	5 large
Yam, baked	65g/2¼ oz
FRUITS	
Apple	2 average
Apricot	5 whole
Banana	1 small
Blueberries	145g/5oz
Figs	2 whole
Grapefruit	1 large
Grapes	25 pieces

Kiwi fruit	3 whole
Mango	1 small
Melon, cantaloupe	½ medium
Nectarines	1 whole, large
Peaches	2 medium
Pears	1 large
Plums	3 whole
Raisins	75 pieces
Raspberries	400g/14oz
Strawberries	300g/10½oz
Tangerines	4 whole
Watermelon	2-cm/1¼-in slice large melon

BREADS AND PASTA

Bagel, plain	⅓ bagel
Garlic bread	1 slice
Malt bread	1 slice
Muffin, mixed berry	½ muffin
Muffin, wholemeal	⅔ muffin
Pasta (recommended serving size is 60g/2oz)	30g/1oz
Raisin bread	1 slice
White bread	1½ slices
White bread, thin	2 slices
Wholemeal bread	1 thick slice
Wholemeal bread, low-calorie	2 slices

CEREALS

All-Bran	40g/1¼oz
Allison Bran Muesli	30g/1oz
Alpen	30g/1oz
Corn flakes	30g/1oz
Frosted wheat	30g/1oz

CARBOHYDRATES	100-CALORIE PORTION

CEREALS (CONT.)

Jordan's Country Crisp	20g/³⁄₄oz
Porridge oats	30g/1oz
Quaker Oat Krunchies	30g/1oz
Rice Krispies	30g/1oz
Sultana bran	30g/1oz
Weetabix	1½ biscuits

CRACKERS

Finn Crisp	3 crackers
Krispen, rye	7 crackers
Ry-King, wheat plus	2 crackers
Ry-King, fibre plus	3 crackers
Ryvita, high-fibre crackerbread	7 crackers
Ryvita, original	4 crackers
Slymbread, original	10 crackers
Slymbread, sesame	7 crackers

SPICES AND CONDIMENTS

Ketchup	60ml/2fl oz
Salsa	180ml/6fl oz
Sugar	6 tsp
Syrup	2 tbsp

FATS	100-CALORIE PORTION

OILS AND SPREADS

Butter	15g (½oz)
Corn oil	2 tsp
Mayonnaise	1 tbsp
Olive oil	2 tsp
Peanut butter	1 tbsp

1,200-CALORIE DAILY MEAL PLANS
FOR THE COUNTING CALORIES DIET

(Dishes in **bold print** are listed alphabetically in the recipe section at the end of the chapter, on page 179.)

DAY

Breakfast

Bran flakes (or some other high-fibre cereal)	130
120ml/4fl oz skimmed milk	40
¼ cantaloupe melon	50
1 slice low-calorie wheat bread	40
1 tablespoon peanut butter	95
Total calories	**355**

AM Snack

1 plum	40
Mini Babybel cheese	60
Total calories	**100**

Lunch

240ml (8fl oz) chicken and rice soup	75
Mixed lettuce salad with tomatoes and cucumbers dressed with 1 tablespoon **Roquefort Soured Cream Dressing**	200
2 Ryvita crackers	56
Total calories	**331**

PM Snack

20g (¾oz) crunchy pretzels	75
Total calories	**75**

Dinner

1 boneless chicken breast 115g (4oz), dredged in ½ Parmesan cheese and ½ bread crumbs, sautéed briefly in olive oil	300
150g (5½oz) asparagus	30
1 tomato, sliced	15
225g (8oz) raspberries with 2 tbsp Anchor Light aerosol cream	80
Total calories	**425**

Total calories for Day 1	**1,286**

DAY

Breakfast

30g (1oz) oats (not instant) with sweetener (not sugar) and 60ml (2fl oz) skimmed milk	125
60g (2oz) blueberries	40
2 slices back bacon	90
Total calories	**255**

AM Snack

1 carton (125g/4½oz) very low fat yoghurt	60
Total calories	**60**

Lunch

120ml (4fl oz) black bean soup	55
2 slices ham on low-calorie bread with lettuce, tomato and 1 teaspoon each mayonnaise and mustard	230
Total calories	**285**

PM Snack

1 raw carrot and 1 stick celery	50
3 tablespoons hummus	105
Total calories	**155**

Dinner

145g (5oz) prawns with 2 tbsp low-calorie mayonnaise	250
1 medium artichoke	15
Sliced tomatoes and cucumbers with 1 tablespoon **Vinaigrette**	75
50g (1¾oz) light vanilla ice cream	89
Total calories	**429**

Total calories for Day 2	**1,184**

DAY 3

Breakfast

Breakfast sandwich (½ muffin, 1 poached egg, 1 slice back bacon, 1 slice processed cheese)	235
¼ cantaloupe melon	50
Total calories	**285**

AM Snack

Sliced cucumbers with 100g (3½oz) low-fat natural cottage cheese	100
Total calories	**100**

Lunch

240ml (8fl oz) cream of asparagus soup (made with water)	85
1 large tomato stuffed with **Tuna and Sweetcorn Salad**	225
Total calories	**310**

PM Snack

2 plums	70
Total calories	**70**

Dinner

Chicken Mediterranean	385
200g (7oz) runner beans	40
Pure fruit juice lolly	60
Total calories	**485**

Total calories for Day 3	**1,250**

DAY

Breakfast

1 slice watermelon	35
1 slice cheese toast with tomato (1 slice low-calorie bread, 2 slices tomato, 1 slice , Gruyère or low-fat Cheddar cheese with a smear of mustard)	130
Total calories	**165**

AM Snack

Small **Fruit Smoothie** (½ serving)	140
Total calories	**140**

Lunch

Open sandwich of low-calorie bread, 115g (4oz) sliced turkey, tomato and lettuce with ½ tablespoon mayonnaise	270
60g (2oz) grapes (approx 12)	30
Total calories	**300**

PM Snack

1 small pack low-fat crisps	130
Total calories	**130**

Dinner

120g (4oz) grilled tuna, seasoned with 3 tablespoons salsa	225
170g (6oz) spinach, sautéed with garlic in spray of olive oil	50
170g (6oz) steamed baby carrots	50
120ml (4fl oz) fruit sorbet	150
Total calories	**475**

Total calories for Day 4	**1,210**

DAY 5

Breakfast

60g (2oz) sultana bran with 120ml (4fl oz) skimmed milk	220
1 slice low-calorie bread with 1 tablespoon peanut butter	135
Total calories	**355**

AM Snack

240ml (8fl oz) turkey vegetable soup	72
Total calories	**72**

Lunch

Greek Salad	190
2 original Ryvita crispbreads	54
¼ cantaloupe melon	50
Total calories	**294**

PM Snack

2 tangerines	50
Total calories	**50**

Dinner

1 serving **Pork Chops with Sweet Potatoes and Apples**	339
1 medium artichoke	15
225g (8oz) raspberries with 2 tablespoons Anchor Light aerosol cream	80
Total calories	**434**

Total calories for Day 5	**1,205**

DAY

Breakfast

Omelette made with 1 whole egg and 2 additional egg whites, and chopped green pepper, onion and tomato	150
½ serving **Ambrosia**	115
Total calories	**265**

AM Snack

2 figs	70
30g (1oz) prosciutto ham	50
Total calories	**120**

Lunch

240ml (8fl oz) clam chowder	80
1 small baked potato stuffed with salsa and 2 tablespoons low-fat soured cream	250
¼ cantaloupe melon	50
Total calories	**380**

PM Snack

12 almonds	70
Total calories	**70**

Dinner

12 medium boiled prawns	65
Cocktail sauce (2 tbsp ketchup mixed with horseradish)	30
1 ear corn on the cob (no butter)	125
1 cup steamed broccoli	35
225g (8oz) sliced strawberries with 2 tablespoons Anchor Light aerosol cream	86
Total calories	**341**

Total calories for Day 6	**1,176**

DAY 7

Breakfast

Fruit Smoothie	280
1 slice low-calorie bread, toasted	40
1 tablespoon peanut butter	95
Total calories	**415**

AM Snack

¼ cantaloupe melon	50
Total calories	**50**

Lunch

Endive and tomato salad dressed with **Avocado Dressing**	245
2 Ryvita crackers	56
1 tangerine	25
Total calories	**326**

PM Snack

20g (¾oz) crunchy pretzels	75
Total calories	**75**

Dinner

115g (4oz) fat-free ham, heated in microwave oven	120
Winter Squash Supreme	280
15 spears asparagus	40
Total calories	**440**

Total calories for Day 7	**1,306**

RECIPES FOR CALORIE COUNTERS

✳

For your convenience, the recipes are listed in alphabetical order.

AMBROSIA

2 oranges, halved
1 banana, sliced
40g (1¼oz) desiccated unsweetened coconut

Peel and thinly slice 3 of the orange halves. In a bowl, combine the sliced oranges, banana and coconut. Juice the remaining orange half and pour the juice over the fruit mixture. Let sit for 5 to 10 minutes before serving.

MAKES 2 SERVINGS
PER SERVING: 230 CALORIES

AVOCADO DRESSING

½ avocado, peeled and mashed
60ml (2fl oz) vinegar
½ teaspoon Dijon mustard
120ml (4fl oz) olive oil

In a small bowl, combine the avocado, vinegar and mustard. Drizzle in the oil while stirring. Mix well. Use immediately.

MAKES 6 SERVINGS (180ML/6FL OZ)
PER SERVING: 180 CALORIES

CHICKEN MEDITERRANEAN

4 tablespoons olive oil

4 chicken legs

1 onion, sliced

1 can (400g/14oz) whole tomatoes

240ml (8fl oz) white wine

1 clove garlic, crushed

Salt

Ground black pepper

Black olives (optional)

Heat the oil in a large saucepan over a medium-high heat. Add the chicken and cook until browned. Remove from the saucepan. Add the onion to the same pan and cook until transparent but not brown. Add the tomatoes, wine and garlic. Add salt and pepper to taste. Add the olives, if using. Replace the chicken in the saucepan. Cover, reduce the heat to low, and cook for 20 minutes, or until the chicken is cooked through.

MAKES 4 SERVINGS
PER SERVING: 385 CALORIES

FRUIT SMOOTHIE

I add a little All-Bran to my smoothies –
I love it; others don't. Try it and see.

240ml (8fl oz) skimmed milk

60ml (2fl oz) natural yoghurt

1 large ripe banana or other soft fruit, such as canned
peaches or fresh or frozen berries

2–3 ice cubes

1 tablespoon All-Bran cereal (optional)

THE COUNTING CALORIES DIET 181

In a blender, combine the milk, yoghurt, banana or other fruit, ice cubes and cereal (if desired). Blend until smooth.

MAKES 1 SERVING
PER SERVING: 280 CALORIES

GREEK SALAD

SALAD

1 head romaine lettuce, washed and shredded, or half a lettuce and 100g (3½oz) spinach

1 medium tomato, cut into wedges

½ small onion, thinly sliced

60g (2oz) low-fat feta cheese, crumbled

6 Greek olives, stoned

DRESSING

60ml (2fl oz) red wine

1 tablespoon olive oil

1 tablespoon dried oregano

2 teaspoons lemon juice

1 teaspoon fresh basil, chopped, or ½ teaspoon dried basil

To make the salad: In a large bowl, combine the lettuce or lettuce-spinach mixture with the tomato, onion, cheese and olives.

To make the dressing: In a small bowl, mix the wine, oil, oregano, lemon juice and basil. Add to the salad and toss to mix.

MAKES 2 SERVINGS
PER SERVING: 190 CALORIES

PORK CHOPS WITH SWEET POTATOES AND APPLES

3 tablespoons plain flour

Salt

Ground black pepper

2 pork chops, 90g (3oz) each

30g (1oz) diced onion

120ml (4fl oz) chicken stock

60ml (2fl oz) cider

1 small sweet potato, sliced

1 apple, sliced

In a shallow bowl, mix the flour with salt and pepper to taste and dredge the pork chops in the flour mixture.

Heat a large non-stick frying pan sprayed with olive oil over a medium-high heat. Add the pork chops and cook for about 2 minutes on each side, or until brown. Remove from frying pan and set aside.

In the same frying pan, combine the onion and a small amount of the chicken stock. Cook until the onions are tender and translucent. Add the cider and the remaining chicken stock. Return the pork chops to the pan, add the sweet potato and apple. Cover, reduce the heat and simmer until the sweet potato and apple are tender.

MAKES 2 SERVINGS
PER SERVING: 339 CALORIES

ROQUEFORT SOURED CREAM DRESSING

115g (4 oz) Roquefort or blue cheese

240ml (8fl oz) low-fat soured cream

1 tablespoon vinegar

1 tablespoon finely chopped onion or chives

Salt

Ground black pepper

In a blender, combine the cheese, soured cream, vinegar and onion or chives. Blend to the desired consistency. Add salt and pepper to taste.

Makes 6 servings
Per serving: 130 calories

TUNA AND SWEETCORN SALAD

150g (5½oz) corn, fresh or frozen, cooked; or canned, drained

1 can (170g/6oz) tuna in brine

3 sticks celery, chopped

½ onion, finely chopped

120ml (4fl oz) low-fat mayonnaise

Red pepper, diced

Salt

Ground black pepper

This recipe tastes best with fresh sweetcorn. Cook it in a microwave oven for 2 to 3 minutes, then cut it off the cob. If using frozen corn, cook it in a microwave oven for 1 minute, then rinse with cold water.

In a bowl, mix together the corn, tuna, celery, onion and mayonnaise. Add the red pepper, salt and pepper to taste.

Makes 4 servings
Per serving: 200 calories

VINAIGRETTE

80ml (3fl oz) olive oil
80ml (3fl oz) wine vinegar
80ml (3fl oz) water
1–2 cloves garlic, crushed
Salt
Ground black pepper

In a small bowl, mix the oil, vinegar, water and garlic. Add
salt and pepper to taste.

MAKES 12 SERVINGS (240ML/8FL OZ)
PER SERVING: 56 CALORIES

✻ *You can replace up to half of the vinegar with mustard –
Dijon mustard works best.*

WINTER SQUASH SUPREME

2 tablespoons olive oil
1 small butternut squash, cut into bite-size chunks
1 apple, cut into bite-size chunks, peeled if you like
115g (4 oz) fresh cranberries
2 tablespoons brown sugar

Heat the oil in a large frying pan over a medium-high heat.
Add the squash and cook, stirring frequently, for 5 to 7 minutes, or until it starts to soften. Add the apple. Cook together
for another 5 minutes, then add the cranberries and brown
sugar. Cook until everything is tender and the cranberries are
swollen and soft.

MAKES 2 SERVINGS
PER SERVING: 280 CALORIES

CHAPTER 8

THE COUNTING FATS DIET

UNTIL VERY RECENTLY, if you went to your doctor and said you wanted to lose weight, he would hand you some pamphlets about a low-fat, high-carbohydrate diet. That was the only eating option offered by doctors, nutritionists and, for many years, even women's magazines. And while many doctors continue to plug the old standby, few books and checkout-counter magazines tout that weight-loss strategy today. Your grandmother's diet could use a good public-relations agent. It's struggling as it competes with the South Beach diet and the Carbohydrate Addict's diet. While there are a dozen different versions of the Atkins diet, low-fat diets, with their exhortations to 'Eat More and Weigh Less' or to 'Stop the Madness' have practically disappeared from magazine covers and faded to the background of bookshop shelves.

So, can you lose weight on a low-fat diet? Or was it, as one recent story in *The New York Times Magazine* proclaimed, 'A Big Fat Lie'? It was no lie. But in the ongoing debate about dieting, it always seems that the new idea disproves the old one. It doesn't, of course, and that's the main point of this book. Each of these fitness regimes works, but it depends on who the dieter is and how well the plan is customized to the individual eater. The fact is, there have been hundreds of studies done on low-fat diets documenting their effectiveness. By one analysis, every 2 per cent drop in the amount of fat you eat is associated with a 450g (1lb) weight loss.

Successful dieters also testify to the effectiveness of a low-fat diet. In a survey of 440 men and women who had lost at least 13.5kg (30lb) and maintained that weight loss for more than 5 years, many swore by a low-fat diet as the strategy they used to lose weight, and for virtually all it was a key component to how they maintain their new weight.

The big problem with the low-fat diet was that, until recently, it was the only diet available. Everybody got put on this diet, regardless of how they ate, how they lived and what made them satisfied. It was the original, the officially sanctioned one-size-fits-all diet.

When that happened, the failure rate for the low-fat diet, of course, soared. Sure, lots of people were able to lose weight, but many more were not. And because it was considered the 'right' way to eat, the failures were even more likely to be seen as a moral failing rather than a simple mismatch between dieter and diet.

Moreover, all fat became the 'enemy'. Because of this new way of thinking, the difference between 'good' fats and 'bad' fats was lost, and the important role that fat plays in any diet was forgotten. As a result, this very effective approach to weight loss has been virtually abandoned – not by doctors and nutritionists, but by dieters who chalk it up to just one more failed diet strategy.

So who is this diet right for? Like all diets, that will depend on your food preferences, the ways in which you get full, your medical history and your lifestyle. To figure out whether you should use a low-fat diet, you'll need to understand the basics of how one works – in other words, which fats to keep, which to get rid of and, perhaps most important, which foods you can use to keep you from missing fats once you cut them down to size. This is the key feature that often makes low-fat diets fail: you must fashion a diet that will help you lose weight and yet allow you to feel satisfied. If you are suffering as you diet, then that diet won't work. Once you understand how a proper low-fat diet works, we'll move to a list of foods containing 5 grams of fat or less and a 7-day eating plan so you can see how to put these principles into action. Finally, at the end of the chapter, I have provided recipes that will give you some fresh ideas on how to cook and eat when you are counting fats.

Let's start with a look at the successful low-fat dieter.

DIANE'S STORY

Diane is an attractive, 44-year-old woman who came to me when it looked to her as if it were inevitable that she would end up as big and round as her mother and her two older sisters. She is almost 1.83m (6ft) tall, and so the weight she carried, just over 90kg (14½ stone), made her look tall and shapely, not at all fat. But over the past several years, her weight kept creeping upwards. Her son, Matthew, now 7, had left her 6.8kg (15lb) heavier than what she thought was her best weight, 72.5kg (11½ stone), and since her separation 2 years before, the scales seemed to move in only one direction. She was frustrated and a little angry.

'It's just not fair,' she told me. 'Okay, I'm not perfect. But mostly I eat right. Sometimes, though, I do eat too much, and when that happens, I feel like I put on the weight and then it just never comes off. It's not fair!'

We talked about her life and her diet. During the week, it was very hectic at her house; frequently, she was too busy to eat breakfast. Those days she might grab a doughnut and coffee after dropping off the kids on the way to work. For lunch, she and the other women at her office went to a neighbourhood deli and got sandwiches – and the tasty homemade crisps that went with them.

Dinner was erratic. The older child liked only sandwiches, and the younger one ate only macaroni cheese. Once the kids were in bed, she often ate dinner standing at the refrigerator, picking at the leftovers from the weekend or from the pasta she made for her daughter. Diane's scheduled meals were small, but what she didn't eat at mealtime she ate (plus a lot more) at snack time. At the office, Diane couldn't usually resist when everyone took a break around 3:00 or 4:00 PM and raided the confectionery machines downstairs. Then after supper, she often rewarded herself with biscuits ('They were lowfat!') when she did the laundry or paid the bills.

We went over her food diary. Lots of pasta, lots of sandwiches, crisps, occasional chicken, occasional sweets. Soft drinks almost daily. I asked her about red meat: she didn't much care for it, and as for trying to get her kids to eat it – no chance.

Her biggest complaint about dieting? Hunger. Usually she dieted by eating only meals and cutting out the snacks, but she noticed that a couple of hours after every meal she'd be famished. One thousand calories, she'd tell herself. She watched the clock for lunchtime and was the first one out the door at 5:30, her stomach growling.

These last few years, every diet ended in disaster. She would lose weight, but after a few weeks the constant hunger and sense of deprivation would wear her down, and she would find herself stuffing herself with any biscuits, crisps or sweets she could find.

The other thing she hated about dieting was never eating enough to really feel full. She measured out her portions oh-so-carefully, but 75g (2½oz) of pasta, wow, it sure didn't look like 250 calories. She liked to limit her meal calories so that she could treat herself with sweets for dessert. Without dessert, she felt she could never stick to a diet, because she would just feel even more deprived. She'd carefully measure out her 80ml (2½fl oz) of ice cream (110 calories), savouring every spoonful. Filled with a feeling of real accomplishment, she could put the box away even when she was dying for more. But it never lasted. 'I just don't have the willpower.'

After our talks and looking over her food diary and questionnaire, I thought Diane would do best on a fat-counting diet. What was it that made her a good candidate? First of all, her food preferences led her there. She ate lots of pasta, breads and veggies. She rarely ate meat, and when she did, it was chicken or occasionally fish. What kept her from having a true low-fat diet were her high-fat snacks. Eating what she thought was a healthy low-calorie diet was making her hungry, and when she was hungry, the yummy treats of her office mates or in her cupboard were too hard to resist.

Even after a meal, she felt that she hadn't really eaten 'enough'. She wasn't really hungry, but she didn't feel really satisfied either. Eating a little of this and a little of that – the essence of a low-calorie diet – seemed silly, and she'd rather sit down to a huge salad than to a plate dotted with small servings of lots of different foods.

So what makes *you* a good low-fat dieter? Like Diane, you need to like the foods that make up a low-fat diet. So carbohydrates are going to play an important role: breads and pastas, fruits and vegetables; these foods make up the cornerstone of a fat-counting diet. You should be on this diet only if you love them. Low-fat proteins will also play an important role. This includes not only low-fat meats such as poultry and fish but also non-meat sources of protein: beans, soya, dairy products and eggs.

How you get full will also contribute to whether or not you do well on a low-fat diet. Volume should be an important satisfaction signal for successful low-fat dieters. It may seem obvious that, of course, everyone needs to have that feeling of fullness in their stomach to stop eating – but that's not true. We all have a variety of cues that tell us we've had enough. If you are reading this chapter, chances are you get your strongest sense of fullness from volume.

Although food preference and satisfaction are the two most impor-

---

WHO SHOULDN'T EAT A LOW-FAT DIET?

You probably shouldn't be on this diet if you have:

- Diabetes
- Metabolic syndrome
- High triglycerides
- Low HDL (good) cholesterol

These conditions suggest that you don't process carbohydrates normally, and carbs are the heart of this diet.

---

tant characteristics in choosing a low-fat diet, other aspects of your health and lifestyle also contribute. The presence of certain cardiac risk factors may have been key in selecting this type of diet for you.

And this diet requires you to eat frequently. Eating three meals per day plus two snacks will be essential for the maintenance of this diet. Let the word go forth: I am 'prescribing' snacks as the cure. Why? Because for many eaters, it's better to graze throughout the day, eating and snacking from time to time to ward off big hunger attacks. Those notorious collapses in the low-fat diet – those moments when you just can't take it any more and you just have to dive head-first into a packet of chocolate chip cookies until it's empty – are the problem. So, strange as this may sound, you have to be willing to eat when you are hungry to enjoy this diet and make it work.

THE BASICS OF A FAT-COUNTING DIET: MORE IS MORE

Fat contains more calories than any other form of food. The purpose of fat in our bodies – and in the bodies of the plants and animals that provide us with our fat – is to store energy. And it does that very well.

A gram of carbohydrates or protein contains 4 calories. A gram of fat contains 9 calories – more than twice as many. That difference lies at the heart of the fat-counting diet. Ultimately, a low-fat diet must be a low-calorie diet for you to lose weight. If you reduce the fat in your diet, while eating the right carbohydrates and proteins, you really can eat more food while taking in fewer calories.

This works because of something we are reminded of every Christmas. One of the most important ways we have of being satisfied by a meal is volume. In very concrete ways, in our stomachs, more is just, well, more. While we have ways of monitoring calories so that we end up eating the same number of calories on a day-to-day, week-to-week basis, our ability to figure the calories in a single meal is remarkably poor. We don't stop eating because we have taken in enough calories. In fact, when we stop eating, most of those calories are lying untouched in our stomachs. What makes us stop is volume. And, in fact, most people eat the same volume of food each day. When researchers have done studies of men and women to see what triggers they have to make them stop eating, volume repeatedly comes out first. In other words, if you eat something that takes up a lot of room in your stomach but doesn't have very many calories, you are going to be more satisfied than if you ate something that didn't take up much room but had lots of calories.

Unfortunately, quantity may fool our stomachs on a single-meal basis – which is how most of these studies are done – but it doesn't always get us from one meal to the next. Eating a head of lettuce will fill you up, but chances are that in an hour or so you will be ready to eat again. Fats (and proteins) play an important role in keeping us feeling full so that we can last more than an hour or two between meals. You have to outsmart your body by keeping some fats and replacing the rest with foods that have fewer calories but can send the same type of powerful message to the brain that you have eaten and that it was good.

JOHN'S STORY

John is a 39-year-old Italian man who started and now runs a family-owned business. He was in pretty good shape when he was younger but began putting on weight after he had a family and started his business. By the time I met John, he was almost 22.6kg (3½ stone) over what he considered to be his best weight. He had high blood pressure, and his knees hurt. He also had sleep apnoea and needed to use a special air pump when he went to sleep every night. His cholesterol levels were out of control. His doctor told him that he would have to start taking medication if he didn't get his LDL cholesterol levels down. He didn't want to take any medicines, but his father had had a heart attack in his fifties and John didn't want that either. That's when he came to see me.

John's days were hectic. He opened the shop at 7:30 each morning and often didn't get home until after 9:00 PM. When he got up in the mornings, he'd jump into the shower and rush off to work. He reported that he usually ate only one meal a day, dinner, because that was really the only meal he was hungry for. He never ate breakfast. Not hungry and no time, he said. If he got a few hunger pangs late in the morning, there was always something to snack on around the office. He rarely stopped for lunch. He might grab a slice of pizza or a bag of fries – whatever the kids in the shop were eating. By the time he ate dinner, he was starving. Sometimes he felt like he ate all night long, from the moment he got home until he went to bed, because he just couldn't get a feeling of really being full.

Like Diane, his diet was primarily carbohydrates. He did eat meat, but usually fish or chicken, and he rarely had milk or butter. Cheese was a staple only because it came with the pizza he ate.

John had been on a diet several years ago. He'd joined Weight Watchers and had lost almost 22.6kg (3½ stone) over the course of the year. He'd tried to put himself back on that diet but had never really got it to work for him. He couldn't stick to it, because he felt hungry all the time.

After reviewing John's history and questionnaire, it seemed clear to me that a fat-counting diet would be best for him. It was right for his taste and temperament, it was right for his health, and it had worked in the past. I thought that John was having trouble making it work since then because he was trying to cut out fats without changing the rest of his diet, and that simply won't work for most people. And when he wasn't dieting, his habit of eating only one meal a day was contributing to the problem. By making him get so hungry that he couldn't keep himself from overeating, his eating habits were part of the problem, not the solution.

John, like many dieters, allowed himself to starve all day long, and when he finally sat down to eat, he was driven to overeat. It's your body's natural reaction to deprivation, and it's as inevitable as gravity. No matter whether you are trying to lose weight or just maintain the weight you have, it's important that you eat when you are hungry, not when you are starving.

That is particularly important on a fat-counting diet. When you eat a diet high in carbohydrates, as you will on a fat-counting diet, you are providing your body with its preferred fuel. That means your body will be able to use these calories right away – and that's good. What that means, though, is that you will need to refuel at regular intervals to keep your body running. That means three meals a day and probably a snack or two. Otherwise, you end up too hungry once you are at the table and, like John, find yourself unable to stop.

THE PERFECT FIT COUNTING FATS BASIC DIET

So what does a fat-counting diet look like? In this eating plan, probably more than any other, you have to think about not only the foods you're avoiding but also the foods you'll be replacing them with. Although the supermarket carries hundreds of low-fat products, many of them may not necessarily be low in calories.

On this diet, you will be eating some fat – up to a third of your calories will come from fats. And the fats you eat will be the 'right' fats – those that are good for you. In addition, you'll be eating lots of naturally low-fat carbohydrates. And you will be eating plenty of protein, because while carbs fill up your stomach, proteins help you feel satisfied and stay that way for hours at a time.

THE LOW-DOWN ON FAT

All fats are not created equal.

The Perfect Fit Counting Fats Diet provides you with about one-third of your calories from fat. This allows you some of the satisfying qualities of fat while reducing your total fat intake.

But it's not just a matter of getting rid of all kinds of fats. A healthy low-fat diet will eliminate the 'bad' fats while increasing the 'good' kind. Most of the fat in the average diet is bad: either saturated

THE HIDDEN COST OF LOW-FAT FOODS

Low-fat versions of foods frequently contain just as many calories – and sometimes even more – than their original version. In taking the fat out, manufacturers often put extra carbohydrates in. For example, low-fat peanut butter has one-third the amount of fat and yet still has around 85 calories per tablespoon.

A standard biscuit made by one company can have fewer calories than the reduced-fat version made by another company. Read the label before you sample any low-fat foods to make sure they are low-calorie as well.

HOW MUCH FAT?

'No diet will remove all the fat from your body, because the brain is entirely fat. Without a brain, you might look good, but all you could do is run for public office.' – *George Bernard Shaw*

How much fat do you need in the diet? We all need some.

• Infants need to get 50 per cent of their calories from fat.

• Children up to the age of 2 should get up to 40 per cent of their calories from fat.

• Adults can get by with 15 to 20 per cent of their calories from fat – if they want to.

fats – those found in meat or high-fat dairy products – or a type known as trans fats. These are the fats that increase risk of heart disease and possibly cancer.

You may not have heard much about trans fats. They are only beginning to get the attention they deserve. These are found naturally in tiny proportions in many foods, but most of the trans fats we eat are made in a laboratory (not that there's anything wrong with that). And though they fit the definition of monounsaturated or polyunsaturated fat, they act just like saturated fats in the body and seem to be linked to higher rates of coronary artery disease. Where do you find these trans fatty acids? Wherever partially hydrogenated oils are sold. These are the fats used in many processed foods – biscuits, breads, pastries. They add a creamy quality to the food and increase shelf life, so manufacturers love them. They also add to your risk of heart disease.

So, on the Perfect Fit Counting Fats Diet, you reduce your intake of saturated fats by eating less meat and then only lean cuts of meat. And you will reduce trans fats by avoiding prepackaged baked goods and other foods containing these fats. Then you replace some of that fat with mono- and polyunsaturated fats – which are derived from nuts, grains and olives – plus omega fats, which are found in seafood.

These healthy fats frequently make up only a small portion of the fat in a typical Western diet. You can eat more of these and still get only 33 per cent of your calories from fat. Because you need to make distinctions among fats, I don't call this a low-fat diet: I call it a fat-counting diet, because you pay attention not just to the fats you get rid of, but to the fats you keep as well.

THE SECRET OF THE COUNTING FATS DIET: KNOW YOUR LABELS

If you are going to pay attention to the fats you eat and reduce your fat to one-third of the calories in your diet, you need to know how to read a food label. Sounds easy, but it can be confusing. The labelling of foods was the result of the pro-consumer movement that emerged in the 1970s, but the food industry managed to influence how the labels got written. So, yes, the information is there, but it's often there in surprisingly deceptive ways – ways meant to trick us into eating (and therefore buying) more.

First, you have to learn the lingo. The law states only that claims should not be misleading. The Food Standards Agency (FSA) recommends that the term 'low fat' should only be used on foods that contain less than 3 grams of fat per 100 grams, and 'fat free' only on foods that contain a tiny amount of fat – less that 0.15 grams per 100 grams. 'Reduced fat' claims should be restricted to foods that contain less than three-quarters of the amount of fat in the standard product (in other words, reduced-fat mayonnaise should have, at most, three-quarters of the fat of normal mayonnaise).

The label will also tell you how many calories are in each serving. Knowledge is power: you need to know how many calories a food has, because it can really surprise you.

Second, the label tells you what a serving is. Often what you might think of as a single serving might not be what is listed as a serving on the label. Alternatively, on some products – particularly fizzy drinks – the label only gives nutritional data per 100ml of the product. So for the standard 500ml bottle of cola that most people would regard as a single serving, you would need to multiply the number of calories listed by five.

The food label will also tell you how much fat is in each serving, and it will list how much of that fat is saturated fat. You want to limit fats in general on this diet to 33 per cent, and you want to limit saturated fats to less than 7 per cent of your total caloric intake.

Here's what's not on the label: what percentage of the calories in

How to Read a Label

Nutrition Information
Typical values

	Per 100g	Per 30g
Energy	2086kJ	626 kJ
	497kcal	149kcal
Protein	7.0g	2.1g
Carbohydrate	7.0g	2.1
of which sugars	19.2g	5.7g
starch	47.8g	14.3g
Fat	22.4g	6.7g
of which saturates	9.8g	2.4g
Fibre	3.0g	0.9g
Sodium	0.6g	0.2g

Always check the serving size – what you consider a serving may not match the manufacturer's idea of a serving.

Check the calories per serving – you may be surprised at what you read.

Here's where the maths comes in. To figure out the percentage of calories from fat, multiply the grams of fat per serving by 9 (the amount of calories in a gram of fat). Then divide the total calories per serving by the calories from fat. In this case $6.7 \times 9 = 60.3$; $149 \div 60.3 = 2.4$. If your answer is less than 3, the food contains too much fat.

Saturated fat should make up no more than 7 per cent of your daily calories. On a 1,200-calorie diet, that's just 9 grams.

the food come from fat. For that you have to do a little maths: fat provides 9 calories per gram so you multiply the number of grams of fat per serving by 9 and then divide the number of calories in the serving by the number of calories from fat. If that number is less than 3, then more than a third of the calories come from fat, and you want to limit how much of that food you eat.

Here's another thing not on the label: how much of the fat is monounsaturated and polyunsaturated fat. You might think you could figure that out simply by subtracting the saturated fats from the total fat and you would end up with the amount of mono- and polyunsaturated fats. But you wouldn't, because manufacturers don't have to list the trans fats. At least not yet. Until they do, you need to look on the panel listing the ingredients, and if you see the phrase 'partially hydrogenated oils', then you know trans fats are in the food, though you won't know the amount.

Now, if I'm not eating fats, what am I eating? If you take away the fats, you are going to be hungrier if you continue to otherwise eat the same way. A diet that restricts fats can work only if you make sure the carbohydrates and proteins that you eat will take over the job of making you feel full with fewer calories.

THE RIGHT STUFF: PROTEIN

Proteins are the backbone of any successful diet. First of all, they are foods that help make you feel full. Carbohydrates alone can't do it. If you neglect your protein, you will feel hungry, and if you feel hungry, you will not be able to maintain your diet. What this means is that every meal and every snack should contain at least a small amount of protein to keep you feeling satisfied and full.

Secondly, your body needs protein every day because body parts (made primarily of protein) have to be repaired, and you have virtually no storage capacity for proteins. So you need to eat proteins every day. When you are restricting calories, your body will turn to muscle for the extra calories to keep running, often before it looks to fat stores. You don't want to lose muscle mass when you lose weight, because muscle helps burn calories. So what's a dieter to do? Eat more protein, say the studies.

Meat is the richest source of protein. Each 30g (1oz) of beef contains 9 to 10 grams of protein. But it's also the form highest in fat – mostly saturated fat. So, on this diet you should look to non-meat sources of protein for much of each day's supply. Dairy products have protein in them: each 240ml (8fl oz) of low-fat milk or yoghurt contains 8 grams of protein; each 30g (1oz) of low-fat cheese has 7 to 8 grams. Starchy beans (like kidney beans or pinto beans, not the green beans you snap) have about 9 grams per 100g (3½oz). How much protein you'll be needing when you are dieting is based on your weight. In general, you should eat about 7 grams of protein for every 4.5kg (10lb) of your current weight. You should try to get your protein from all the different classes of foods on a low-fat diet.

For example, a 68kg (10st 10lb) woman should eat 35 grams of protein each day. She'd get that with 480ml (16fl oz) of semi-skimmed milk (remember, it goes in your coffee and your cereal), a carton of low-fat yoghurt or cottage cheese, a serving of three-bean salad, a string cheese stick and 90g (3oz) of lean meat.

A 90kg (14¼-stone) man would get enough protein with 480ml (16fl oz) of semi-skimmed milk, a poached egg, a slice of back bacon, a container of yoghurt, a handful of nuts, 115g (4oz) of fish, a serving of rice and beans and a scoop of frozen yoghurt. That's a lot of food.

I don't want you to feel as if you have to go around counting your protein. It's hard enough just keeping track of the fat. But I do want you to get an idea of just how much protein we need to keep our bodies running well and our bellies full.

THE RIGHT STUFF: CARBOHYDRATES

Carbohydrates will continue to make up the largest category of foods you eat on a fat-counting diet. Like meat, carbohydrates can come attached to large amounts of fat. This is especially true of carbs you

10 TIPS TO REDUCE YOUR FAT INTAKE

1. Limit your total fat intake to one-third of your total calories consumed in a day.

   • On a 1,500-calorie diet, this means 55 grams of fat.

   • On a 1,200-calorie diet, this means 44 grams of fat.

2. Limit your saturated fat intake to less than 7 per cent of your total calorie intake.

   • On a 1,500-calorie diet, this mean only 12 grams of saturated fat.

   • On a 1,200-calorie diet, this means only 9 grams of saturated fat in a given day.

3. To do this . . .

   • Limit red meat such as beef to one or two meals per week, and when you eat it, cut off visible fat.

   • Avoid ground meats – even those marked 'extra lean' contain more fat than a T-bone steak.

   • Remove the skin from poultry.

   • Roast, grill or bake when you can.

   • If you need to cook in fat, sauté in olive oil.

   • Limit portions to 90 to 115g (3 to 4oz) at each meal.

   • Avoid ready-prepared foods.

4. Limit butter and avoid margarine altogether. Margarine doesn't taste as good as butter and, because of the trans fatty acids, is just as bad for you. (There are some buttery spreads with no trans fats.)

don't prepare yourself. Fats are often added to packaged foods in order to beef up the taste and lengthen shelf life. On this diet, you need to avoid prepackaged foods and go back to basics. This means not buying frozen meals or canned or frozen prepared foods. You

5. Use only skimmed milk and low-fat or fat-free cheeses.

6. Eat seafood as often as you can. It does have fat (though usually much less than beef), but it has virtually no saturated fat and is loaded with omega fatty acids, which still have lots of calories, but can reduce your risk of heart disease.

7. Plan your meals around a carbohydrate and use the fat-containing foods as a flavour ingredient rather than as the focus of the meal.

8. When you eat eggs, use fewer yolks than whites. The yolks contain all the cholesterol, and a 2:3 or even 2:4 ratio of egg yolks to egg whites is just as flavoursome with much less fat and cholesterol.

9. Replace high-fat foods with low-glycaemic-load carbohydrates plus some protein whenever possible. Instead of snacking on a bag of crisps, eat a piece of fruit or vegetable with a low-fat cheese or yoghurt, or dip your veggies in hummus.

10. Eat vegetarian for one or two meals per week. Vegetarian cuisine is filled with foods that make you feel full while limiting fat intake. Vegetarian meals use a wide variety of beans and grains that provide the protein and low-glycaemic-load carbohydrates that make up a healthy and satisfying low-fat diet.

11. (An extra) Try different seasonings. Fat is an easy way to add flavour to foods, but there are many sauces and flavouring strategies that can provide just as much flavour with virtually no fat. (I've given some ideas for flavouring low-fat meats, seafood and vegetables in the recipe section at the end of this chapter.)

might be thinking, 'Oh, I just don't have time for that!' I understand, but many of the foods that make up a fat-counting diet don't take any longer to prepare than microwavable TV dinners, they are better tasting and, let's face it, much better for you.

The carbohydrates you eat on the Perfect Fit Counting Fats Diet, like the fats you eat, need to be the right variety. Some carbohydrates will make you feel full and satisfied. Others will leave you craving more – if not right away then in an hour or two. How can you distinguish between the right carbs and the wrong ones? Researchers have come up with a system to help you do just that called the glycaemic load. Foods with a low GL will help you feel full, while those with a high GL will make you feel hungry. (For a list of common foods and their glycaemic loads, see page 129.)

Generally, low-GL foods include fruits, vegetables and foods made from whole grains. These are what many people call 'whole foods', that is, foods that have not been processed – foods we eat pretty much as they come. High-GL foods are usually foods that have been refined. Think of foods made from white flour, like breads, biscuits and pastries. Can this make weight loss easier? Research says yes: eating a diet packed with low-GL foods has been shown to help people lose weight at least in part by making them feel full for longer.

Does the Counting Fats Diet work? It does for people who like to eat this way. Let's go back to Diane. She started a low-fat, low-glycaemic-load diet and went from 92 to 82kg (14½ to 13 stone) in 4 months. As hard as it was, she made a point of eating breakfast with her kids every day. And she started taking in her lunch every day to work. She was worried that she would feel left out when the other women went to the corner deli, but most of them started bringing in their lunches too. It gives them a lot more time to sit and talk. She also began exercising every day. She told me that she'd never before felt so good. She's continued to lose weight, although not nearly as quickly. She now weighs 75kg (11¼ stone). She's still not at her target, but she's getting there. Her sister was so intrigued by Diane's success that she started on the diet as well. Now they are exercising together every day.

And what about John? It was tough initially, but he's eating three meals a day, and just doing that has made him feel a lot better. The office is still filled with the kind of food he doesn't want to eat despite his attempt to ban them. He brings in his own snacks, however, and that goes a long way towards keeping him satisfied so that most days he can walk past the pizza without stopping. He lost 9kg (20lb) in his first 3 months on his diet and has gone back to practising his tae kwon do almost every day. His blood pressure is down and so is his cholesterol.

What does a low-fat, low-glycaemic-load diet look like? To help you put these theories into practice, I have provided a list of foods in quantities that contain 5 grams of fat or less, a 7-day meal plan and some tasty low-fat recipes.

THE PERFECT FIT COUNTING FATS DIET: THE BIG PICTURE

- Reduce total fat to 33 per cent of your calories.
- Eat the right fats by avoiding saturated and trans fats while enjoying mono- and polyunsaturated fats and omega fats.
- Eat the right carbohydrates by replacing processed, high-glycaemic-load foods with whole, low-glycaemic-load carbs.
- Include a low-fat protein in every meal and snack to help you feel full longer.

FOOD LIST FOR COUNTING FATS BASIC DIET

These low-fat foods in the amounts listed contain 5 grams of fat or less. (Calories for portion sizes are also included. These are based on typical single-serving sizes.)

FOOD	AMOUNT	CALORIES
VEGETABLES		
Artichoke	Unlimited	15 per globe
Asparagus	Unlimited	30 per 10 spears
Aubergine	Unlimited	15 per 100g/3½oz
Avocado	⅙ small fruit	67 per ⅙ fruit
Beans, baked	170g/6oz	145 per 170g/6oz
Beans, butter	Unlimited	77 per 100g/3½oz
Beans, kidney	Unlimited	105 per 100g/3½oz
Beetroot	Unlimited	46 per 100g/3½oz
Black-eyed peas	340g/12oz	116 per 100g/3½oz
Broccoli	Unlimited	24 per 100g/3½oz
Brussels sprouts	100g/3½oz	35 per 100g/3½oz
Cabbage	Unlimited	16 per 100g/3½oz
Carrots	Unlimited	31 per large carrot
Cauliflower	Unlimited	28 per 100g/3½oz
Celery	Unlimited	7 per 100g/3½oz
Chickpeas	170g/6oz	86 per 75g/2½oz
Corn on the cob	3 ears	125 per large ear
Courgette	10 large	18 per 100g/3½oz
Cucumbers	8 whole	34 per cucumber
Lettuce (all varieties)	Unlimited	5 per 30g/1oz
Mushrooms	Unlimited	5 per mushroom
Onion	Unlimited	36 per 100g/3½oz
Peas, green	Unlimited	117 per 170g/6oz
Peppers, fresh	5 medium	25 per large fruit
Potato	Unlimited	200 per large potato
Potato, sweet	Unlimited	130 per large potato
Radishes	Unlimited	2 per large radish
Soya beans	100g/3½oz	141 per 100g/3½oz

Spinach	Unlimited	7 per 30g/1oz
Squash, acorn	Unlimited	39 per 75g/2½oz
Squash, butternut	Unlimited	22 per 75g/2½oz
Tomato, canned	Unlimited	40 per 250g/9oz
Tomato, fresh	Unlimited	17 per large fruit
Yam	Unlimited	133 per 100g/3½oz

FRUITS

Apples	Unlimited	80 per fruit
Apricots	Unlimited	12 per fruit
Bananas	7 large	120 per fruit
Blueberries	1.8kg/4lb	64 per 100g/3½oz
Cantaloupe melon	Unlimited	50 per ¼ fruit
Cherries	Unlimited	40 per 100g/3½oz
Coconut	15g/½oz	67 per 15g/½oz
Grapefruit	Unlimited	15 per ½ fruit
Grapes	1.1kg/2½lb	30 per 60g/2oz/ approx 12 grapes
Kiwi fruit	8 fruits	45 per large fruit
Mango	8 fruits	135 per large fruit
Olives	5 medium	46 per 5 medium olives
Oranges	10 medium	65 per large fruit
Pears	7 medium	60 per large fruit
Plums	7 large	36 per fruit
Prunes	Unlimited	20 per large fruit
Raisins	Unlimited	135 per 50g/1¾ oz
Raspberries	Unlimited	16 per 65g/2¼ oz
Strawberries	Unlimited	27 per 100g/3½oz
Watermelon	685g/1½lb	31 per 100g/3½oz

MEAT, POULTRY AND SEAFOOD (All meats are trimmed of visible fat.)

Beef

Beef brisket	30g/1oz	179 per 90g/3oz
Beef sirloin	75g/2½oz	168 per 90g/3oz
Chuck and blade	170g/6oz	179 per 90g/3oz

FOOD	AMOUNT	CALORIES
MEAT, POULTRY, AND SEAFOOD (CONT.)		
Skirt	60g/2oz	176 per 90g/3oz
Topside	90g/3oz	180 per 90g/3oz
Lamb		
Lamb chop	50g/1¾oz	190 per 90g/3oz
Leg of lamb	50g/1¾oz	183 per 90g/3oz
Pork		
Bacon, streaky	1½ slices	125 per 3 slices
Bacon, back	3 slices	90 per 2 slices
Ham	90g/3oz	124 per 90g/3oz
Pepperoni	2 slices	27 per slice
Pork chop	60g/2oz	182 per 90g/3oz
Pork loin	90g/3oz	165 per 90g/3oz
Pork sausage	½ sausage	110 per sausage
Poultry		
Chicken, dark meat, no skin	45g/1½oz	225 per 115g/4oz
Chicken, white meat, no skin	115g/4oz	175 per 115g/4oz
Turkey, dark meat, no skin	75g/2½oz	175 per 115g/4oz
Turkey, white meat, no skin	200g/7 oz	176 per 115g/4oz
Turkey sausage	2 links	46 per link
Seafood		
Clams	320g/11oz	133 per 90g/3oz
Cod, Atlantic	Unlimited	89 per 90g/3oz
Crab	100g/3½oz	115 per 90g/3oz
Flounder	350g/12oz	83 per 90g/3oz
Haddock	340g/12oz	80 per 90g/3oz
Lobster	300g/10½oz	118 per 115g/4oz
Mussels	100g/3½oz	94 per 90g/3oz
Oysters	250g/9oz	61 per 90g/3oz
Prawns	500g/1lb 2oz	90 per 90g/3oz

Salmon, canned	75g/2½oz	138 per 90g/3oz
Salmon, fresh farmed	45g/1½oz	175 per 90g/3oz
Swordfish	90g/3oz	132 per 90g/3oz
Trout	90g/3oz	120 per 90g/3oz
Tuna, canned in brine	400g/14oz	90 per 90g/3oz
Tuna, fresh	500g/1lb 2oz	97 per 90g/3oz

CHEESE

Cheddar, low-fat	30g/1oz	82 per 30g/1oz
Cottage cheese	115g/4oz	120 per 115g/4oz
Cottage cheese, low-fat	145g/5oz	90 per 115g/4oz
Cream cheese, light	30g/1oz	60 per 30g/1oz
Feta	20g/¾oz	75 per 30g/1oz
Gruyère	15g/½oz	120 per 30g/1oz
Mozzarella, light	30g/1oz	56 per 30g/1oz
Parmesan	15g/½oz	125 per 30g/1oz
Processed, light	1⅓ slice	45 per slice
Ricotta, light	60g/2oz	39 per 30g/1oz
String cheese	30g/1oz	80 per 30g/1oz

DAIRY

Cream, light single	45ml/1½fl oz	57 per 45ml/1½fl oz
Egg, cooked omelette style	½ egg	88 per egg
Egg, hard-boiled	¾ egg	88 per egg
Egg white from 1 egg	Unlimited	12 per egg
Egg yolk from 1 egg	1 egg	61 per egg
Frozen yoghurt, fat-free	Unlimited	100 per 120ml/4fl oz
Ice cream, vanilla	60ml/2fl oz	140 per 120ml/4fl oz
Ice cream, vanilla, reduced fat	180ml/6fl oz	100 per 120ml/4fl oz
Light choc ice	1 bar	100 per bar
Milk, skimmed	1.2 litres/2 pints	80 per 240ml/8fl oz
Milk, semi-skimmed	300ml/10fl oz	114 per 240ml/8fl oz

FOOD	AMOUNT	CALORIES
DAIRY (CONT.)		
Milk, whole	150ml/5fl oz	163 per 240ml/8fl oz
Soured cream	1 tbsp	40 per 1 tbsp
Soured cream, half-fat	2 tbsps	30 per 1 tbsp
Yoghurt, very low-fat	Unlimited	100 per 240ml/8fl oz
Yoghurt, low-fat, fruit-flavoured	350ml/12 fl oz	200 per 240ml/8fl oz
Yoghurt, low-fat, natural	240ml/8fl oz	145 per 240ml/8fl oz
FATS AND OILS		
Butter	5g/1 tsp	111 per 1 tbsp
Hummus	1½ tbsp	33 per 1 tbsp
Margarine	5g/1 tsp	111 per 1 tbsp
Margarine, reduced fat	10g/2 tsp	83 per 1 tbsp
Margarine, half-fat	15g/½ oz	55 per 1 tbsp
Mayonnaise	½ tbsp	100 per 1 tbsp
Mayonnaise, light	1 tbsp	42 per 1 tbsp
Olive oil	1 tsp	99 per 1 tbsp
Vegetable oil	1 tsp	99 per 1 tbsp
NUTS AND SEEDS		
Almonds	10g/⅓oz	183 per 30g/1oz
Brazil nuts	10g/⅓oz	205 per 30g/1oz
Cashews	10g/⅓oz	183 per 30g/1oz
Macadamia nuts	2 nuts	224 per 30g/1oz
Pecans	7g/¼oz	207 per 30g/1oz
Pine nuts	7g/¼oz	206 per 30g/1oz
Pistachio nuts	10g/⅓oz	180 per 30g/1oz
Sunflower seeds	approx 15 seeds	174 per 30g/1oz
Walnuts	approx 4 halves	206 per 30g/1oz

BREADS, GRAINS, AND PASTA

Bread, light	Unlimited	40 per slice
Bread (most varieties)	5 slices	80 per slice
Muffin (not sweet)	2 muffins	140 per muffin
Pasta (raw, dried)	285g/10oz	210 per 30g/1oz
Popcorn	15g/½oz	110 per 20g/¾oz
Rice, brown	340g/12oz (cooked)	140 per 100g/3½oz (cooked)
Rice, white	340g/12oz (cooked)	140 per 100g/3½oz (cooked)
Rice, wild	Unlimited	163 per 50g/1¼oz
Rice cake, wholegrain	17	28 per cake
Taco shells	1 shell	98 per shell
Wheat germ	60g/2oz	108 per 30g/1oz

CEREALS

All-Bran	125g/4½oz	108 per 40g/1¼oz
Luxury fruit muesli	75g/2½oz	150 per 40g/1¼oz
Oats	60g/2oz	110 per 30g/1oz
Sultana bran	150g/5½oz	128 per 40g/1½oz
Weetabix	170g/6oz	143 per 2 biscuits

BISCUITS AND CRACKERS

Choc-chip cookie	2 x 10g cookies	47 per cookie
Cream cracker	2 crackers	30 per cracker
Oatcake	2 oatcakes	54 per oatcake
Semi-sweet rich tea type	3 biscuits	35 per biscuit

BEVERAGES

Coca-Cola	Unlimited	149 per 350ml/12fl oz
Coffee	Unlimited	5 per 240ml/8fl oz
Diet Coke	Unlimited	2 per 350ml/12fl oz
Ginger beer	Unlimited	152 per 350ml/12fl oz
Juices	Unlimited	100 per 240ml/8fl oz
Soya milk	240ml/8fl oz	81 per 240ml/8fl oz

DAILY MEAL PLANS FOR THE COUNTING FATS DIET

(Dishes in **bold print** are listed alphabetically in the recipe section at the end of the chapter, on page 218.)

DAY

	Fat (g)	Calories
Breakfast		
30g/1oz high-fibre cereal (bran flakes)	0.5	95
120ml/4fl oz semi-skimmed milk	2	55
125g/4½oz fresh berries	0	30
1 slice low-calorie, high-fibre bread	0.5	40
1 tablespoon peanut butter	8	95
Total fat and calories	**11**	**315**
AM Snack		
2 tablespoons hummus	3	70
Sliced celery and carrots	0	50
Total fat and calories	**3**	**120**
Lunch		
240ml/8fl oz black bean soup	1.5	115
1 ripe tomato, sliced	0	25
40g/1¼oz reduced-fat mozzarella cheese, sliced	4	75
2 tablespoons chopped fresh basil	0	0
Vinaigrette	5	42
Ryvita crispbread, 2 crackers	0	56
Total fat and calories	**10.5**	**313**
PM Snack		
240ml/8fl oz very low fat yoghurt	0	100
Total fat and calories	**0**	**100**

Dinner

	Fat (g)	Calories
Lemon Chicken Cutlets	10	300
75g/2½oz brown rice	1	110
170g/6oz broccoli, steamed and served with lemon	0	45
Total fat and calories	**12**	**455**
Total fat and calories for Day 1	**37**	**1,303**

DAY

	Fat (g)	Calories
Breakfast		
20g/¾oz oats (not instant – these have a much higher glycaemic load) with 120ml/4fl oz skimmed milk and 1 teaspoon sugar	2	135
¼ cantaloupe melon	0	50
1 slice low-calorie bread, toasted	0.5	40
1 tablespoon peanut butter	8	95
Total fat and calories	**10**	**320**
AM Snack		
String cheese stick	5	80
1 medium apple	0.5	60
Total fat and calories	**5.5**	**140**
Lunch		
Black and White Bean Salad	3	175
4 Ryvita slimmers' crispbread	1	112
Total fat and calories	**4**	**287**
PM Snack		
1 pure fruit juice lolly	0.5	60
Total fat and calories	**0.5**	**60**

Dinner

	Fat (g)	Calories
Chicken and Vegetable Bake	6	207
Romaine lettuce, tomatoes and artichoke hearts	1	100
Vinaigrette	5	42
125g/4½oz strawberries	0.5	34
2 tablespoons Anchor Light aerosol cream	2	25
Total fat and calories	**14.5**	**408**
Total fat and calories for Day 2	**36**	**1,215**

DAY

	Fat (g)	Calories
Breakfast		
3-egg omelette using 2 yolks and 3 whites, filled with chopped onion, green peppers and tomato	10	250
½ grapefruit with 1 teaspoon sugar	0	35
Total fat and calories	**10**	**285**
AM Snack		
Grapes (approx 2 dozen)	0.5	80
Total fat and calories	**0.5**	**80**
Lunch		
240ml/8fl oz chicken vegetable soup	1.5	90
Vegetable Sandwich	16.5	280
Total fat and calories	**18**	**370**
PM Snack		
15g/½oz plain popcorn	1	75
Total fat and calories	**1**	**75**

Dinner

	Fat (g)	Calories
1 serving **Pork Chops with Sweet Potatoes and Apples**	7	339
10 stalks asparagus steamed, seasoned with lemon	0	30
Small fresh salad with **Vinaigrette**	5	100
Total fat and calories	**12**	**469**
Total fat and calories for Day 3	**41.5**	**1,279**

DAY 4

	Fat (g)	Calories
Breakfast		
30g/1oz high-fibre cereal (bran flakes)	0.5	95
120ml/4fl oz semi-skimmed or 180ml/6fl oz skimmed milk	2	55
75g/2½oz fresh berries	0	20
2 slices back bacon	4	90
Total fat and calories	**6.5**	**260**
AM Snack		
3 Ryvita-type slimmers' crispbreads with 50g (1¾oz) low-fat cottage cheese	1.5	120
Total fat and calories	**1.5**	**120**
Lunch		
Ham and Gruyère sandwich with lettuce and tomato on low-calorie bread with mustard	12	255
Carrot sticks	0	50
Total fat and calories	**12**	**305**

PM Snack

	Fat (g)	Calories
1 large apple	0.5	80
Total fat and calories	**0.5**	**80**

Dinner

	Fat (g)	Calories
115-g/4-oz tuna steak, grilled, topped with **Pico de Gallo**	1.5	140
1 medium artichoke, steamed and dipped in **Vinaigrette**	5	60
115g/4oz butter beans, steamed	0.5	85
120ml/4fl oz frozen yoghurt	5	150
Total fat and calories	**12**	**435**
Total fat and calories for Day 4	**33**	**1,200**

DAY 5

	Fat (g)	Calories
Breakfast		
Fruit Smoothie	2	280
1 slice low-calorie bread, toasted	0.5	40
2 tablespoons hummus	3	70
Total fat and calories	**5.5**	**390**

	Fat (g)	Calories
AM Snack		
1 stick celery, ½ raw carrot and 60g/2oz broccoli florets	0	50
Total fat and calories	**0**	**50**

Lunch

Greek Salad	13	190
1 small pitta bread	0.5	75
Total fat and calories	**13.5**	**265**

PM Snack

Grapes (about 2 dozen)	0.5	80
Total fat and calories	**0.5**	**80**

Dinner

Beef Stroganoff	17	380
200g/7oz broccoli florets	0	48
1 pure fruit juice lolly	0.5	60
Total fat and calories	**17.5**	**488**
Total fat and calories for Day 5	**37**	**1,273**

DAY

	Fat (g)	Calories
Breakfast		
3-egg omelette using 2 yolks and 3 whites, filled with chopped onion, green peppers and tomato	10	250
2 slices lean back bacon, grilled	4	90
½ grapefruit with 1 teaspoon sugar	0	35
Total fat and calories	**14**	**375**
AM Snack		
1 large pear	0	50
Total fat and calories	**0**	**50**

Lunch

	Fat (g)	Calories
240ml/8fl oz clam chowder	2	80
Ham and Gruyère sandwich with lettuce and tomato on low-calorie bread with mustard	12	255
Total fat and calories	**14**	**335**

PM Snack

15g/½oz plain popcorn	1	75
Total fat and calories	**1**	**75**

Dinner

Boiled prawns (about 20 large)	2	100
2 tbsps Cocktail sauce (ketchup and horseradish)	2	30
1 corn on the cob (no butter)	0	125
Small salad with 2 tablespoons **Green Goddess Dressing**	3	90
1 light choc ice	5	100
Total fat and calories	**12**	**445**
Total fat and calories for Day 6	**41**	**1,280**

DAY

	Fat (g)	Calories
Breakfast		
Eggs Carbonara	17	262
½ cantaloupe melon	0	100
Total fat and calories	**17**	**362**

AM Snack

240ml/8fl oz very low-fat yoghurt	0	100
Total fat and calories	**0**	**100**

Lunch

Tuna and Sweetcorn Salad	12	192
3 Ryvita-type slimmers' crispbreads	0.5	80
Total fat and calories	**12.5**	**272**

PM Snack

1 pure fruit juice lolly	0.5	60
Total fat and calories	**0.5**	**60**

Dinner

Ratatouille	15	223
Grilled chicken breast 115g/4oz	3.5	140
75g/2½oz steamed mangetout	0	20
125g/4½oz strawberries topped with 2 tablespoons Anchor Light aerosol cream	2.5	59
Total fat and calories	**21**	**442**

Total fat and calories for Day 7	**51**	**1,236**

RECIPES FOR FAT COUNTERS

⁎

For your convenience, the recipes are listed in alphabetical order.

BEEF STROGANOFF

4 tablespoons plain flour

Salt

Ground black pepper

340g/12oz rump or skirt steak, cut into strips

4 tablespoons olive oil

2 cloves garlic, crushed

170g/6oz sliced onions

2 green peppers, sliced

90g/3oz sliced mushrooms

240ml/8fl oz fat-free beef stock

455g/1lb low-fat natural yoghurt

455g/1lb cooked noodles

In a shallow bowl, mix 3 tablespoons of the flour with salt and black pepper to taste and dredge the steak in the flour mixture. Heat the oil in a large frying pan over a medium-high heat. Add the steak and cook, stirring frequently, for about 5 minutes, or until brown. Add the garlic, onions and peppers and cook for 2 minutes, stirring frequently. Add the mushrooms and cook for another 2 minutes, stirring frequently. Add the beef stock and bring the mixture to the boil. Cover, reduce the heat and simmer for 10 minutes.

Meanwhile, in a small bowl, mix the soured cream and the remaining flour. Stir until smooth, then add into the simmering mixture. Cook for about 2 minutes, stirring frequently, until the mixture is thickened. Serve over noodles.

MAKES 4 SERVINGS
PER SERVING: 17G FAT, 380 CALORIES

BLACK AND WHITE BEAN SALAD

1 can (400g/14oz) black beans, rinsed and drained

1 can (400g/14oz) cannellini beans, rinsed and drained

120ml/4fl oz cider vinegar

1 tablespoon olive oil

1–2 cloves garlic, finely chopped

½ teaspoon chilli flakes

2 large ripe tomatoes, chopped

1 medium onion, chopped

1 green or red pepper, chopped

2 sticks celery, chopped

2 large carrots, chopped

6 tablespoons chopped parsley

12 stoned olives, chopped

Salt

Ground black pepper

Romaine lettuce or fresh spinach

In a large bowl, combine the black beans, cannellini beans, vinegar, oil, garlic and chilli flakes. Mix and set aside as you chop the tomatoes, onion, pepper, celery, carrots, parsley and olives. Mix the vegetables with the beans and add salt and black pepper to taste. Serve on a bed of romaine lettuce or fresh spinach.

MAKES 6 SERVINGS
PER SERVING: 3G FAT, 175 CALORIES

✳ *You can substitute white or brown rice for the cannellini beans.*

✳ *If you can't find black beans in the shops substitute borlotti beans.*

CHICKEN AND VEGETABLE BAKE

1 tablespoon olive oil

1 small onion, chopped

2 sticks celery, chopped

1 green pepper, chopped

115g (4oz) sliced carrots

170g (6oz) sliced fresh mushrooms

455g (1lb) chicken breasts, cut into small pieces

115g (4oz) frozen green peas (see note)

240ml (8fl oz) low-fat chicken stock

3 tablespoons flour

Heat the oil in a large non-stick frying pan over a medium-high heat. Add the onion, celery, pepper and carrots and cook, stirring frequently, until the vegetables begin to soften. Add the mushrooms and cook, stirring frequently, until soft. Add the chicken and peas and cook, stirring frequently, until the chicken is lightly browned. Pour into a casserole dish.

In a small bowl, whisk 3 tablespoons of the chicken stock with the flour to form a smooth paste. Add the remainder of the chicken stock and stir until thickened. Pour into the baking dish with the chicken and vegetables.

Bake at 180°C (350°F), gas 5 for 20 to 25 minutes.

MAKES 5 SERVINGS
PER SERVING: 6G FAT, 207 CALORIES

✳ *Frozen green peas are almost as good as fresh and a lot handier.*

EGGS CARBONARA

1 teaspoon butter

3 egg whites

2 egg yolks

90g (3oz) lean ham, diced

60g (2oz) frozen peas, thawed

40g (1¼oz) Parmesan cheese

In a non-stick frying pan, melt the butter. In a small bowl, beat together the egg whites and egg yolks. When very fluffy, pour into the frying pan. Cook over a low heat until the edges are firm.

Heat the ham in a microwave oven. Add the ham and peas to half of the eggs, and fold the other half over. Cook until the top is firm. Sprinkle with the cheese before serving.

MAKES 2 SERVINGS
PER SERVING: 17G FAT, 262 CALORIES

FRUIT SMOOTHIE

I add a little All-Bran to my smoothies –
I love it; others don't. Try it and see.

240ml (8fl oz) semi-skimmed milk

60ml (2fl oz) natural yoghurt

1 large ripe banana or other soft fruit, such as canned peaches or fresh or frozen berries

2–3 ice cubes

1 tablespoon All-Bran cereal (optional)

In a blender, combine the milk, yoghurt, banana or other fruit, ice cubes and cereal (if desired). Blend until smooth.

MAKES 1 SERVING
PER SERVING: 2G FAT, 280 CALORIES

GREEK SALAD

SALAD

1–2 heads lettuce, washed and shredded, or half lettuce
    and half spinach

1 medium tomato, cut into wedges

½ small onion, thinly sliced

60g (2oz) low-fat feta cheese, crumbled

6 Greek olives, stoned

DRESSING

60ml (2fl oz) red wine

1 tablespoon olive oil

1 teaspoon dried oregano

2 teaspoons lemon juice

2 teaspoon chopped fresh basil or ½ teaspoon dried basil

To make the salad: In a large bowl, combine the lettuce or lettuce-spinach mixture with the tomato, onion, cheese and olives.

To make the dressing: In a small bowl, mix the wine, oil, oregano, lemon juice and basil. Pour the dressing over the salad and toss to mix.

MAKES 2 SERVINGS
PER SERVING: 13G FAT, 190 CALORIES

GREEN GODDESS DRESSING

240ml (8fl oz) low-fat natural yoghurt

2 tablespoons low-fat mayonnaise

2 teaspoons lemon juice

1 teaspoon vinegar

1 clove garlic, finely chopped

2 tablespoons chopped parsley

½ teaspoon English mustard

1 teaspoon chopped fresh tarragon or ½ teaspoon dried
tarragon

In a small bowl, combine the yoghurt, mayonnaise, lemon
juice, vinegar, garlic, parsley, mustard and tarragon. Mix well.

Makes 8 servings
Per serving: 3g fat, 40 calories

LEMON CHICKEN CUTLETS

3 tablespoons flour

Salt

Ground black pepper

2 chicken breasts

1 tablespoon olive oil

1 lemon, thinly sliced

1 tablespoon capers

60ml (2fl oz) white wine

In a shallow bowl, mix the flour with salt and pepper to taste.
Dredge the chicken breasts in the flour mixture.

Heat the oil in a non-stick frying pan. Add the chicken and
cook for about 5 minutes, turning it over to make sure it
cooks through. Take the chicken from the frying pan and set
aside. In the same frying pan, combine the lemon and capers.
Cook until the lemon rinds are soft, then remove the lemons
and add the wine. Simmer until the sauce has reduced by
half, about 8 to 10 minutes. Return the chicken to the frying
pan. Lower the heat and simmer together for 3 to 5 minutes.

Makes 2 servings
Per serving: 10g fat, 300 calories

PICO DE GALLO

455g (1lb) tomatoes, peeled, seeded and coarsely chopped

8 spring onions, finely chopped

1 jalapeño pepper, finely chopped (wear plastic gloves when handling) or chilli flakes

2 tablespoons lime juice

1 clove garlic, finely chopped

Salt

Ground black pepper

3 tablespoons chopped fresh coriander leaves

In a bowl, combine the tomatoes, spring onions, jalapeño or desired amount of chilli flakes, lime juice and garlic. Add salt and black pepper to taste. Stir in the coriander. Refrigerate 1 hour before serving.

MAKES 6 SERVINGS
PER SERVING: 0.5G FAT, 17 CALORIES

PORK CHOPS WITH SWEET POTATOES AND APPLES

3 tablespoons plain flour

Salt

Ground black pepper

2 pork chops, 90g (3oz) each

60g (2oz) diced onion

120ml (4fl oz) chicken stock

60ml (2fl oz) apple cider

1 small sweet potato, sliced

1 apple, sliced

In a shallow bowl, mix the flour with salt and pepper to taste and dredge the pork chops in the flour mixture.

Heat a large non-stick frying pan sprayed with olive oil over a medium-high heat. Add the pork chops and cook for about 2 minutes on each side, or until brown. Remove from the frying pan and set aside.

In the same frying pan, combine the onion and a small amount of the chicken stock. Cook until the onions are tender and translucent. Add the cider and the remaining chicken stock. Return the pork chops to the pan, add the sweet potato and apple. Cover, reduce the heat and simmer until the sweet potato and apple are tender.

MAKES 2 SERVINGS
PER SERVING: 7G FAT, 339 CALORIES

RATATOUILLE

2 large aubergines, cut into 1-cm (½-in) thick slices

4 red or yellow peppers, cut into strips

4 large ripe red tomatoes, cored, peeled, seeded and cut into thick slices

2 large onions, thinly sliced

5 cloves garlic, coarsely chopped

½ teaspoon dried thyme

Salt

Ground black pepper

60ml (2fl oz) virgin olive oil

In a 32.5 × 23cm (13 × 9in) baking dish, layer half of the aubergines, peppers, tomatoes and onions. Add the garlic and thyme. Add salt and black pepper to taste. Top with the other half of the vegetables. Drizzle the dish with the oil. Bake for 1 hour at 180°C (350°F), gas 4.

MAKES 4 SERVINGS
PER SERVING: 15G FAT, 223 CALORIES

TUNA AND SWEETCORN SALAD

125g (4½oz) corn, fresh or frozen, cooked; or canned, drained

1 can (170g/6oz) brine-packed tuna

3 sticks celery, chopped

½ onion, finely chopped

120ml (4fl oz) low-fat mayonnaise

Red pepper, diced

Salt

Ground black pepper

This recipe tastes best with fresh sweetcorn. Cook it in a microwave oven for 2 to 3 minutes, then cut it off the cob. If using frozen sweetcorn, cook it in a microwave oven for 1 minute, then rinse with cold water.

In a bowl, mix together the sweetcorn, tuna, celery, onion and mayonnaise. Add red pepper, salt and pepper to taste.

MAKES 4 SERVINGS
PER SERVING: 12G FAT, 192 CALORIES

VEGETABLE SANDWICH

2 slices low-calorie bread

½ very ripe avocado

¼ cucumber, peeled and sliced

½ tomato, sliced

¼ onion, very thinly sliced

¼ green pepper, sliced

1 handful bean sprouts

1 tablespoon Jerusalem artichoke relish

On 1 slice of the low-calorie bread, spread the meat of the avocado. Layer with the cucumber, tomato, onion and pepper. Add the bean sprouts and relish. Top with the second slice of bread.

MAKES 1 SERVING
PER SERVING: 16.5G FAT, 280 CALORIES

✳ *For the Jerusalem artichoke relish, you may substitute any vegetable relish you like or Pico de Gallo (page 224).*

VINAIGRETTE FOR FAT-COUNTING DIET

60ml (2fl oz) olive oil
80ml (3fl oz) wine vinegar
80ml (3fl oz) water
1–2 cloves garlic, crushed
Salt
Ground black pepper

In a small bowl, mix the oil, vinegar, water and garlic. Add salt and pepper to taste.

MAKES 12 SERVINGS (240ML/8FL OZ)
PER SERVING: 5G FAT, 42 CALORIES

✳ *You can replace up to half of the vinegar with mustard – Dijon mustard works best.*

PART

TAILORING YOUR PERFECT FIT DIET TO YOUR TASTES AND TO YOUR LIFE

OKAY. YOU'VE ALREADY DONE ALL THE HEAVY LIFTING: You've kept an eating and exercise diary, and you've filled out the questionnaire. You've scored it and found out which basic diet works best for you. It's time to customize that diet based on what you know about yourself.

Part 4 is broken up into chapters that correspond to sections in the questionnaire, which are cross-referenced to page numbers within these chapters, so you can find the information relevant to your dieting profile. These chapters will give you all the guidance you need to tailor your diet based on everything that you have learned about yourself and about nutrition.

The first chapter in part 4 (chapter 9) deals with the types of foods you prefer, with tips on how to work your favourite kinds of foods into your basic diet. Are you a Carnimore? Are you a Vege-carian? A Starch Stealer? A Sweets Eater? You will find out how to work with these preferences in your diet to achieve the weight you want.

Chapter 10 deals with your dieting history and what makes you feel full and satisfied. Are you someone who needs to eat a certain volume of food in order to feel full? Do you find yourself bored by the foods you are allowed to eat? Do you crave variety? Do you have a hard time feeling full if you haven't eaten something rich, like meat or another source of protein? These are all characteristics of the ways we feel full. We all have these three satiety mechanisms at work, but for many of us, one predominates. Which one is most important to you? Assessing how past diets have worked or not will help you determine which type of cues rule your system.

Chapter 11 evaluates how your medical history and your family's may affect which diet is going to work best for you. Are you a binge eater? Do you have high blood pressure or diabetes? Do you smoke? Your diet should be based on food preference and what makes you feel full, but how your body works is also an important factor. What good is a diet if it makes you feel worse because it's incompatible with other problems in your body? This section addresses those issues.

No man (or woman) is an island, wrote John Donne nearly 400 years ago, and it remains true today. We are individuals, but we come from families, and we carry with us remnants of those origins throughout our lives – in our bodies and in our psyches. Chapter 12 looks at how our genetic and emotional heritage affects the way we look and eat and feel.

It's not just what you eat but *how* you eat it that determines how well a diet will work for you. Do you skip meals frequently? Do you snack when you are bored? Are you a stress eater? Do you overeat at parties? Eating habits can contribute mightily to difficulties you have in maintaining the weight you desire. In chapter 13, I'll address some bad eating habits and offer strategies for modifying them.

Then, in chapter 14, we look at your lifestyle and how it may contribute to the difficulties you have in losing weight or maintaining your optimal weight. Do you eat out more than you eat in? That's a problem, because restaurants tend to load your plate with fattening foods. Do you work so many hours that any non-work activity – eating and exercising included – is squeezed out of your life? Are you chronically sleep-deprived? These are barriers to your being able to achieve and maintain an optimal weight. We'll identify your blocks to weight loss and maintenance and discuss some ways of over-coming them.

Let's get started on designing a programme to work just for you.

CHAPTER 9

FOOD PREFERENCES

CARNIMORE

'Red meat is not bad for you. Now blue-green meat, that's bad for you!'
— TOMMY SMOTHERS, COMEDIAN

If your score was greater than 20 on the Meat and Eggs portion of the questionnaire, then you are probably a Carnimore, that is, someone who enjoys eating meat. Despite its bad reputation, there is nothing wrong with making meat part of your diet and plenty of things right with doing so, but as with everything else in life, there are better and worse ways to do this.

When you think about meat as nutrition, you are really thinking about two fundamental food categories: protein and fat. Let's talk about each of them separately, and then – because we do not eat food components but food itself – we'll put it all back together with recommendations on how to eat meat in a way that is healthy.

Protein: The Good News

Here, in a nutshell, is why protein is so important.

- Protein is the basic building block of all of our body structures and most of the messengers that make our bodies work.
- Meat provides complete proteins that contain all of the amino acids we need to manufacture more proteins that keep our bodies running.
- A diet rich in protein protects muscle mass when you are losing weight.
- Protein intake promotes bone growth. Weight loss causes bone loss, but research has shown that eating a diet that has up to 450 calories a day of protein will help decrease bone loss associated with losing weight.
- Protein makes you feel full. Many studies have been done on the so-called sating effect of foods – that is, how satisfied different foods make you feel – and when fats, carbs and proteins are compared, proteins make you feel full quicker and longer. That's another big plus.

So how much protein do we need? Well, 97 per cent of the population would get enough protein if they ate only 0.3 gram of protein for every 455g (1lb) of body weight. If you look at this in terms of food, it translates into one 170g (6oz) steak if you weigh 68kg (10 stone 10lb). That's per day. That's all.

You Carnimores are probably howling at this point. Remember, that's the minimum. What's the optimal level? The current thinking is that those who are limiting their calories to lose weight should eat at least 0.7 gram per 455g (1lb) of body weight, about double the minimum amount recommended.

So, are you Carnimores who eat more than the allotted protein in trouble? The Harvard Nurses' Study looked at protein intake and risk of heart disease and found that the women who took in the most protein – 25 per cent of their calories every day – had a lower risk of heart disease than women who ate the least amount of protein – an average of 15 per cent per day. And even the lowest consumers of meat still ate considerably more than the minimum.

So, why not go on an all-protein diet?

Protein: The Bad News

Some diets focus on proteins, primarily as a way to reduce carbohydrate intake. These diets, which are very hot right now, want you to replace your pasta and sandwiches with just the meaty toppings and fillings. Any recent fashion magazine is likely to have a story about a model or starlet who has lost weight by eating only meat or fish. It seems to work for many – so, to quote an old burger ad, Where's the beef?

The biggest flaw is this: we doctors worry about the kidneys. Proteins are broken down to their smaller units, amino acids, and those are used throughout the body. Your body can't store protein, so if you eat more than you use, the leftovers have to be broken down and eliminated. It's eliminated, in part, by the kidneys, and the concern is that a diet too high in protein could strain your kidneys.

In laboratories, researchers have watched what happens to the body after a high protein load. Four hours afterwards, more blood is directed to the kidneys, which suggests that they are working harder. So, does working harder definitely mean hurting? Not necessarily, at least not for healthy kidneys. But people who have significant kidney disease should not eat a high-protein diet. And since protein is also broken down in the liver, those with significant liver disease do not do well on a high-protein diet either.

But since you are likely to be eating a diet high in protein, Carnimore that you are, you need to make sure you have enough water in your system to keep your kidneys working well as they get rid of waste. This is one of the major reasons everyone is always told to drink a lot of water – and it is particularly true for Carnimores. Eight glasses of water every day should do the trick.

The other issue for you meat eaters is what you *aren't* getting when you eat nothing but proteins: fibre, vitamins and antioxidants. These are the components of foods that make food good for you. All three are necessary for good health, and these three in particular also prevent disease – including heart disease and cancer. Most protein sources are sorely lacking in these three dietary components, yet no diet is complete without them.

The final problem with a diet that depends too completely on protein has nothing to do with the protein itself and everything to do with another food component frequently linked to it: fat. You know the story here, and you know I'm not saying that all fat is evil. The fact of the matter is that saturated fats, which are the predominant fat in meats, are linked to high cholesterol and heart disease.

Cholesterol and Heart Disease

How does a diet high in saturated fat cause high cholesterol? It's not known exactly, but here's the theory: when we eat fat and cholesterol, it goes to the liver. Then it's shipped around to the places it needs to go in our bodies by little 'taxi' proteins – the most important of which are known as LDL. Something about saturated fats makes it harder for these LDL taxis to deliver the fat to the cells where it's needed. This means the LDL and its fat and cholesterol cargo spend a lot more time in the blood vessels where they're not supposed to be. Eventually, the LDL taxis just dump their load right there and not inside the cells where it belongs. A layer of fat forms on the inside walls of the vessels. This fat layer becomes the foundation for atherosclerosis (hardening of the arteries), and that contributes to heart disease. Trans fats probably work the same way.

Unsaturated fats don't have this problem. They are easily taken up by cells. They don't cause atherosclerotic disease and may actually work to reduce the damage caused by saturated fats. How? A diet high in mono- and polyunsaturated fats gives us more of a different kind of fat taxi known as HDL cholesterol. HDL is known as the good cholesterol because it doesn't deliver fat, it retrieves fat. This tiny taxi goes out into the body and collects excess cholesterol from the arteries and cells and brings it back to the liver where it can be used as energy or shipped out for storage.

And what about omega fats? How are they good for you? When these fats are used to build cells, they make them stronger and less likely to be damaged. It's damage to artery cells that causes heart attacks, so eating a lot of omega fats can make you less likely to get heart disease. Carnimores who eat fish and grass-fed beef (most British beef is grass-fed but beef served in US-based chain restaurants may be corn-fed) may end up with high levels of HDL (good) cholesterol, and that will protect them from heart disease.

What about Eggs?

If cholesterol is the link between saturated fats and heart disease, aren't eggs, which are chock-full of cholesterol, bad for you? Way back in the 20th century, weren't we directed to avoid cholesterol-containing foods – like eggs? Yes, we were, but that connection was probably due to a simplistic understanding of how our bodies work. Cholesterol is a very important substance. Many of our hormones are made of cholesterol – testosterone and oestrogen being two of the most familiar – but cortisol, adrenaline and other very essential hormones are also made from it. Our bodies can make cholesterol, but we also get it through diet. If you eat less cholesterol, you make more of it. If you eat more, you make less. The concern comes when you eat too much cholesterol.

Back when researchers were first investigating the link between

cholesterol and heart disease, it seemed clear that lowering cholesterol was one way to decrease risk of heart disease. And it seemed
reasonable that limiting intake of dietary cholesterol would help
people lower their total cholesterol. Reasonable, but not true. It's one
of the wonders of our bodies that things that seem absolutely logical,
given what we know, don't turn out to be right. So it was with cholesterol. As the case against saturated fats became clearer, the role of
dietary cholesterol became less clear. Was having a high dietary cholesterol level really linked with increased risk of heart disease independent of saturated fat? Well, as it turns out, probably not. And
eating eggs does not seem to increase risk of heart disease.

Of course, there's been a study looking at this. Published in 1999
in the *Journal of the American Medical Association*, this study followed
the course of hundreds of thousands of people who ate eggs. Some
ate them daily, some weekly, some monthly. It was clear that eating
up to seven eggs per week, even over years, did not increase their
risk of heart disease – so it probably won't increase yours either.

That's not that surprising when you know how much good stuff
is in an egg. Eggs are low in saturated fats, high in monounsaturated
fats, high in protein and high in calcium, B vitamins and vitamin A.
The cholesterol is found exclusively in the yolk; the white is mostly
protein. So we welcome the egg back to a healthy diet with open
arms – and mouths.

Carnimores on a low-carb diet who like eggs may find themselves eating more than seven eggs per week. If that sounds like you,
try combining one egg yolk with two egg whites to increase the protein and decrease the cholesterol.

Eating Meat and Eggs: The Plan

So, what's a Carnimore to do?

Here's my advice: go ahead and eat eggs, meat or fish once or twice a day. But – there's always a but, isn't there? – give yourself a good variety of these foods. Specifically, limit your saturated fats and try to eat more fish and seafood.

How much saturated fat is allowed? The current recommendation in the UK is that no more than 10 per cent of energy intake should come from saturated fatty acids. However, this figure is intended as a population average therefore I feel it more appropriate to aim for seven per cent, which is the figure used in the US. Seven per cent. So if you were eating a 1,200-calorie diet, that would allow you 9 grams of saturated fat. If you eat 1,500 calories, you can have 12 grams of saturated fat (7 per cent of 1,500 = 105; this is then divided by 9, the number of calories in a gram of fat).

Tips for Carnimores, No Matter What Diet You Are On

1. Use lower-fat cuts. These are usually cuts such as loin or top-side. The fancier stuff often has a higher fat content: roasts, sirloin and organ meats for example. And skip the ground meats – if you need it, buy a regular cut and have it ground for you.

2. Remember that, in general, beef has more saturated fat than most cuts of pork, which has more fat than most poultry, which has more saturated fat than most types of seafood.

3. When you use lower-fat cuts of meat, they can be a little dry. Don't cook them too long (a meat thermometer helps), and consider adding a little salsa or other low-fat sauce to the meat to boost the flavour.

4. Try lower fat, free-range meats. Free-range chickens, for example, have less fat overall and less saturated fat. And

although they tend to be expensive, they're much tastier and healthier for you.

5. When you cook the meat, make sure you do not add to the saturated fat by adding butter. Cuts or varieties that need added fats should be cooked with olive oil.

FAT CONTENT OF COMMON MEATS

Type of Meat	Fat (g per serving)	Saturated Fat (g per serving)	Notes
Beef	9	5	Trimmed cuts obviously have somewhat less, and fancy cuts (sirloin, etc.) and organ meats have more. Ground beef, even the 'lower-fat' varieties, has the most fat of all.
Lamb	6	2	Legs have less, chops have more. Ground lamb contains up to twice as much fat as the regular cuts.
Pork	7	3	Low-fat cuts (back bacon and ham) can contain as little as 1 gram per serving.
Chicken (skin removed)	4	1	If you eat the skin, add another 2 grams of fat.
Fish (most fish and seafood)	1–2	Less than 1	–
Fish – high fat: includes salmon, mackerel, sardines	5–10	3	In general, wild fish contain 5 grams of fat; farm-bred fish contain twice as much fat.

6. Eat seafood as often as you can. Omega-3 fatty acids are linked to lower cardiac risks. When you eat seafood, choose wild fish over farm-bred fish when you can. The wild variety is much lower in fat. Plus, mercury and PCBs and all the other chemicals we worry about in fish are even lower in the wild types.

7. Portion is learned. So when you crave a steak or some other form of meat, measure your portion; 90 to 115g (3 to 4oz) may look small to you, because you have been trained to expect a 230g (8oz) or even a 340g (12oz) steak. Don't let your eyes talk you into a bigger piece of meat because it's what you are used to. Teach yourself a new portion size. Figure out what you want, not what advertisers tell you that you want.

For carbohydrate counters: Eggs contain virtually no carbohydrate and so are a perfect food for this diet. They do, however, contain some saturated fats and lots of cholesterol. Where possible, consider using one yolk with two whites when you need to cook with eggs. The yolk contains all the cholesterol and most of the calories; the white is mostly protein.

For calorie counters: Mostly because of the fat, meat tends to have a high calorie count. This is where portion control becomes essential. Try buying cuts of meat that are naturally small. For instance, use chicken or turkey fillets or pieces rather than chicken breasts. Lamb chops, while high in fat, are small, and one or two tiny ones may fill your need for meat. Beef comes in thin cutlets too. They have a variety of names; where I live they are called minute steaks. Utilizing these tricks, you won't have to use willpower to maintain your portion control.

For fat counters: If eating red meat only once or twice a week seems like a hardship, try working in small amounts of meat more often. A serving is usually 90 to 115g (3 to 4oz). Try dividing those

small portions into even smaller portions and eating meat more frequently. You can make a great-tasting roast beef sandwich loaded
with tomatoes, lettuce, onions, horseradish and whatever else you
like, using only 30g (1oz) of meat. Or try adding a small amount of
meat to a vegetable stir-fry to reduce the amount of meat in your diet
without making you feel deprived.

KNOW YOUR FATS

Fats can be lumped into two groups: the 'bad' fats, which increase
your risk of heart disease, stroke and some cancers; and the 'good'
fats, which can reduce those risks.

THE BAD FATS

- Saturated fats: These are found primarily in meats and dairy
  products. That white stuff at the edge of your steak – that's it.

- Trans fats: These fats are found in many margarines and shorten-
  ings and provide a smooth, creamy texture to many biscuits,
  crackers and pastries on the supermarket shelf. While they are
  not yet listed on the nutrition label, you can find them in the
  ingredients list as 'partially hydrogenated fatty acids'. When you
  see that ingredient, stay away.

THE GOOD FATS

- Monounsaturated fats: These are most abundant in olive oil and
  rapeseed oil. They are also found in all nuts and in some high-fat
  foods from the fruits and vegetables group, such as avocado.
  Small amounts are also found in lean meats and fish.

- Polyunsaturated fats: These are found in most vegetable oils –
  corn oil, peanut oil, sunflower oil – and in nuts.

- Omega fats: These are most abundant in fish and seafood. They
  are also found in flaxseed, walnuts and their oils.

Use recipes that incorporate meat as an ingredient in a dish rather than featuring meat as the centrepiece of your meal. Where possible, reduce by one-half the amount of meat that's called for in regular recipes.

DAIRY QUEEN OR KING

'Things are seldom what they seem, Skim milk masquerades as cream.'
— SIR WILLIAM SCHWENK GILBERT, *HMS PINAFORE*

Dairy Products: The Good News

If you have a score greater than 50 on the Dairy Products section of the questionnaire, you are likely a Dairy Queen or King – someone who likes butter, cheese and milk in their diet.

The world of nutrition has had mixed feelings about milk over the past couple of decades and, as a result, milk, which used to be considered the very epitome of a health food, is now viewed with some suspicion. In the 1950s and before, the model was the four food groups, so milk and dairy products were touted as foods that should be eaten every day.

Then in the 1970s and 1980s, researchers started looking into sources of cholesterol and saturated fat in the diet, and it was clear that for many people butter, cheeses and whole milk were as impor- tant a source of these dietary demons as red meat. So, we were advised to eschew butter and replace it with margarine. The advice with respect to milk was to avoid it as much as possible, and if you couldn't avoid it, then to make sure that the milk that you drank was skimmed – a greyish, watery liquid, difficult to enjoy after the rich whiteness of whole milk.

If you look at the current government recommendations, you'll find dairy products near the skinny top of the pyramid along with other foods that may be in your diet in small amounts. How the mighty have fallen. Over the past couple of years, these recommendations have started to lose some of their standing, and at this point, it looks as though dairy products should be returning to the fabulous food groups that make up our daily fare.

So, what good comes from dairy products? A lot. First and foremost, for those of us who want to live to a ripe old age, dairy products are an important source of dietary calcium, and calcium is important for the protection of our bones. Since weight loss in and of itself causes bone loss, it's especially important that you do what you can to build up bone mineral density. Research shows that drinking milk is a good way to do that.

Eating dairy products has other health benefits as well. For example, diets rich in dairy products lower blood pressure and reduce the risk of stroke. Diets high in dairy products have also been linked with lower rates of colon cancer. Most compelling is research that suggests that people who eat a high level of dairy products are less likely to be overweight than those with lower intakes. This may be related to an associated decrease in consumption of soft drinks, one of the most common sources of sugar in our diet. But there is evidence that milk and other dairy products contain something that promotes less weight gain – although what, exactly, is not clear.

Finally, some very preliminary research shows that humans, like many animal species, may have a specific appetite for calcium that expresses itself through food preferences. Some very interesting data suggest that calcium supplements decrease the salt cravings that torment so many women before their periods.

Dairy Products: The Bad News

As with all things nutritional, there is also a downside – milk products contain high levels of saturated fats. And many people are lactose intolerant. There are degrees of lactose intolerance, and if you're lucky, then lactase pills might work for you. These can cover you if you really want a pizza with cheese or an occasional ice cream.

Those with significant lactose intolerance, who get the symptoms when they even *think* about milk, should remember that some milk products, like yoghurt, can be eaten without developing symptoms, because they bring their own bacteria. Also, remember that only cow's milk causes the problem. Milks and cheeses from other animals don't. Soya products, while they don't have the same type of benefits as dairy products, have their own plusses. If soya milk and soya ice cream taste good to you, dig in.

Tips for Dairy Queens and Kings, No Matter What Diet You Are On

1. If you are going to drink milk and can't bear the taste of the greyish fluid known as skimmed milk, buy semi-skimmed milk. It has about 1 gram of fat per 100ml (3½fl oz) (so about 20 per cent of its calories come from fat) and only 10 calories more than the skimmed version. It also tastes and looks about a million times better. If you use milk in your coffee, you'll also end up using less of it if you use semi-skimmed milk instead of skimmed.

2. When you are cooking with cheese, you can usually substitute reduced-fat cheeses without affecting the flavour of the dish.

3. Limit your intake of high-fat cheeses, but when you do eat them, eat a moderate amount and try to reduce the amount of fat in the other parts of your diet that day.

4. Use butter just for flavouring, and when you use it, do it sparingly. You might try spreadable butter instead of the usual block stuff. It's easier to use less.

5. Use reduced fat creams instead of regular; the taste is still pretty good.

6. Substitute low-fat or fat-free frozen yoghurt for the ice cream you crave.

For carbohydrate counters: Don't use fat-free dairy products. In general, fat is replaced with carbohydrates in these foods, and dairy products are no exception. On the other hand, lower-fat versions of many of these foods often have an acceptable amount of carbohydrate in them. Check out the label.

For calorie counters: If you like your yoghurt flavoured, buy low-fat or light yoghurt in the smallest containers. These usually contain around 170g (6oz) of yoghurt and give you enough to enjoy while limiting your portion.

For fat counters: The fat in milk and dairy products is mostly saturated and the stuff you want to limit the most. So always use the low-fat version of your favourite dairy product. If they seem thin or

CALORIE, FAT AND CARB CONTENT
OF ORDINARY CHEESES

Cheese	Calories	Fat (g)	Carbohydrate (g)
Cottage cheese, low-fat, 90g (3oz)	90	1–5	4
Feta cheese, 30g (1oz)	75	6	1
Low-fat, soft 60g (2oz)	72	4	2
Mozzarella, whole milk, 30g (1oz)	80	6	1
Mozzarella, reduced-fat, 30g (1oz)	72	3	1
String cheese, 30g (1oz)	80	1	5

watery to you, try stepping down the fat content one step at a time. For example, if you drink whole milk, switch to semi-skimmed, which looks and tastes virtually the same as whole. Then move to skimmed milk. You'll probably be surprised to find you get used to it fairly quickly and more fatty milk tastes overly rich.

VEGECARIAN

'Don't be afraid to go out on a limb – that's where the fruit is.'
— FATHER ANDREW SDC

If you scored higher than 40 on the Fruits and Vegetables portion of the questionnaire, then you may very well be what I call a Vege-carian, and that's wonderful. Fruits and vegetables are good for you and should be at the heart of just about any diet. This is one of the few things most nutrition buffs and diet docs agree on.

Fruits and Vegetables: The Good News

Your mother has been harping on about the benefits of fruits and veggies since you were a kid, so you may not think it's possible for me to come up with any new information on this front. Let me give it a shot.

Fruits and vegetables are a low-calorie, high-nutrient-value food. A diet high in fruits and vegetables will promote weight loss, because these foods contain plenty of water and not so many calories. This is particularly important for those of you who need a lot of food to feel full.

Let me introduce you to the idea of energy density. Basically, that's how many calories a food contains per unit of volume. As it turns out, for many of us, how much food we eat is an important aspect of feeling full. Eating foods with a low energy density allows us to eat satisfying portions of food and still take in fewer calories. Barbara Rolls, PhD, a researcher at Pennsylvania State University, made an important observation a few years ago – an observation that may seem obvious but had never been demonstrated before: most of us eat about the same volume of food each day. What makes up that volume changes from day to day, but the amount stays pretty stable. What this means is that if you eat the same volume but consume fewer calories, you will feel full but will lose weight.

So, what kinds of foods have lower energy density? Generally, these are foods with a high water content, so fruits and vegetables are front and centre. Let me give you an example of how this works: you eat a bowl of pasta for dinner. A 60g (2oz) serving of pasta – that's just over 200 calories – and a light sprinkling of olive oil and Parmesan cheese – that's another 200 calories – and there you have a small serving of pasta. Your 400-calorie meal is tiny, and unlikely to seem the 'right' size to you. But what if you decided instead to add some fresh tomatoes to the pasta – you could sauté the tomato in the olive oil you were going to add to your pasta anyway, then maybe you'd add some onions, courgettes and mushrooms. You could double the amount of food you eat, triple it even, and add fewer than 50 calories. But, chances are, you'd feel a lot fuller after the second dish than the first dish. (Of course, that's a fake argument because you'd probably eat a larger serving of that first one anyway!) Adding vegetables contributes to your sense of satiety without contributing to calories. Now, that's a bargain.

Fruits and veggies are high in fibre, and fibre promotes weight loss. As you know, fruits and vegetables have lots of fibre. At its most basic level, fibre is the stuff in fruits and vegetables that isn't starch and that's hard to digest. There are two kinds of fibre, and they are both good for you, albeit in different ways. Soluble fibre turns to jelly in your stomach. As such, it promotes a sense of fullness, and it slows the absorption of sugar and other nutrients so that your glucose level has less of a tendency to get out of hand. Soluble fibre is found in foods like oats. Diets high in soluble fibre have been found to decrease the risk of heart disease.

Insoluble fibre cannot be absorbed by the gut. It passes through your digestive system virtually untouched. But it promotes stool bulk and causes water to be absorbed by the lower intestines, moving food through and preventing constipation. This is important to everyone, but especially those on a carbohydrate-counting diet, since constipation is a frequent side effect. High-fibre diets reduce the risk of some cancers and help prevent diverticular disease.

Finally, fruits, vegetables and other high-fibre foods may help you lose weight by increasing your body's production of a hormone called protein YY. When obese and thin people are given injections of this protein (as explained in a recent study published in *The New England Journal of Medicine*), they ate much less food over the next 24 hours. Researchers believe that a high-fibre diet, which increases your protein YY level, will also make you feel less hungry.

Fruits and vegetables promote weight loss. Because fruits and vegetables have a lower energy density than most other foods, eating these foods rather than something else will promote weight loss. And most fruits and vegetables are very low glycaemic-load foods, so they not only provide bulk with fewer calories, but they are easy on your insulin level as well, which may help you lose weight too.

There are, of course, exceptions to this rule. Potatoes have a high glycaemic load (GL). One serving of a baked potato has a GL of 26. Much higher that the GL of peas (3), carrots (2) or cherries (3). That puts it in the same category as some cakes and biscuits. Does this mean you can't have potatoes? No, but it means that you should limit your potato intake, and when you do eat them, add a low-fat protein to slow down the glycaemic load. Low-fat cottage cheese does a nice job. Other low-fat cheeses work as well. Or add some salsa with or without a touch of olive oil. And, of course, lower your intake of chips. Most fast-food varieties are fried in oils high in trans fats, so they are a double nutritional debit.

Beta-carotene and other antioxidants prevent disease. You know these are good for you, but do you know why? The way your body is damaged and ages is through oxidation, a perfectly natural process. (On the other hand, so is dying. So if we can fight it, we should.) Dietary antioxidants in the form of fruits and vegetables look like one way to do just that. In one study, people who ate at least five servings of these foods a day lived longer (and were thinner) than those who ate less. But you can't take the healthy ingredients and put them in a pill and get the same benefit. Studies have shown that antioxidant supplements will *not* provide the same protection as their fruit and vegetable sources.

Vitamins and minerals are essential for health. Carbohydrates, proteins and fats are the basic categories of foods that we eat; they are called macronutrients, because they are the energy and building blocks of our bodies. In many foods there are other important components that we call micronutrients. We need only tiny amounts of these components, but they are important for many of the biological processes that go on in our bodies. We need all of these micronutrients, and when we don't get them, we get sick. Many of these come from the fruits and veggies you eat.

Some of the ways fruits and vegetables are treated reduces their nutritional value. Canned foods have lower nutritional value than frozen foods. Frozen foods have lower value than fresh foods. Some ways of cooking are better than others. For example, boiling foods can leach some of the nutrients into the water, which is discarded. Steaming or sautéing avoids this problem. On the other hand, eating these foods any way you can get them is better than not having them, so don't let availability or cooking preference interfere with your eating them.

A special word about nuts: Nuts are not usually considered in a chapter about fruits and vegetables, but I would argue that they ought to be. Nuts are a nutrient-dense food that I think should be made part of a healthy diet. Yes, they are high in calories, they are also high in fibre, high in high-quality protein and high in polyunsaturated fats.

Studies have shown that a diet high in nuts can improve lipids and reduce the risk of heart disease and diabetes. And although nuts have lots of calories and usually lots of salt, they are also high in their ability to sate appetite. (So, eat nuts but avoid bingeing on them.)

How Much Is Enough?

The usual recommendation is to eat five servings of fruits or vegetables per day. I would go further than that. If you like these foods, this group is the one type of food that I would say 'more is better'. These low-glycaemic-index fruits and vegetables can and should be eaten freely. So five servings per day is a good goal, but if you want more, eat more, unless you're on the 30-gram Counting Carbohydrates Diet. Those who are limiting their carbs to 30 grams or less a day will get only a few servings of vegetables and fruits per day. But, remember, that stage of the diet is only for a couple of months. Any longer than that and it becomes much less effective. So the ban on fruit and veggie gorging is brief.

Is There Any Bad News about Fruits and Vegetables?

No. Not from my perspective. Some people are concerned about increasing their exposure to the pesticides used in growing these foods. Within the past 10 years, there has been a great deal of literature published on the subject, particularly in Europe, and the UK Comittee on the Toxicity of Chemicals in Food, Consumer Products and the Environment (COT) has concluded that the probability of any health hazard is likely to be small. These studies have also shown either no or small residues on foods. I think the strongest argument for the healthiness of fruits and vegetables lies in the studies showing that people who eat more fruits and veggies are healthier (not to mention thinner) than those who eat fewer. So, if you like these foods, eat up!

Tips for Vegecarians, No Matter What Diet You Are On

1. Aim for at least five servings of vegetables and four servings of fruit per day.

2. Buy fresh vegetables whenever you can. Only use the canned or frozen stuff when what you want isn't available fresh.

3. When choosing a fruit or vegetable for a snack, make sure you pair it up with a protein to make the snack last. Far too often, people will snack on an apple or carrots several hours before they plan to eat a meal and then find they are hungry an hour or two later. Eating a protein with your carb will give the snack the staying power you need to get you to your next meal without hunger. On the opposite page I have listed some low-fat snacks that add up to 200 calories or less.

For carbohydrate counters: Getting your fill of vegetables and fruits is going to be tough in the early phase of your Counting Carbs Diet, when both serving size and variety are extremely limited. It's easy to eat just a simple salad with your favourite dressing every day. But if you do that, you'll be so bored that it will be hard for you to eat even the limited amount you're allowed. Try different salad dressings to liven up your salad. Most are low in carbohydrates. Also, don't just steam the other veggies. Try sautéing vegetables with a tiny bit of olive oil. Add garlic, chilli peppers and stock or white wine.

LOW-FAT SNACK COMBINATIONS

Snack	Calories	Fat (g)	Carbohydrate (g)
Cantaloupe with 240ml (8fl oz), fat-free plain yoghurt	146	0.2	25
Cucumber (1), sliced, and 2 tbsp hummus	97	3.4	11
Jelly, sugar-free, 50g (1¾oz)	150	0	8
Peach (1), sliced, with 120ml (4fl oz) low-fat cottage cheese	158	1.1	21
Popcorn, butter-flavoured, 15g (½oz)	60	2	12
Potato crisps, baked, 30g (1 oz)	110	5	23
Seven-grain bread, 1 slice, with yeast extract	105	21	1.2
Tomato (1), large, with 30g (1oz) string cheese	118	5.4	7

Casseroles that use eggs and cheese with veggies make a nice change as well. Recipes that show you how to cook the low-carb way can be found at the end of chapter 6.

For calorie counters: Look for new and interesting fruits and vegetables to add to your repertoire. One of the biggest problems with the way many of us eat veggies is boredom. Be adventurous – try new foods and new recipes often. You can start with the recipes at the end of chapter 7.

For fat counters: Rather than slathering your veggies with butter, try other sauces and flavours to spice up the same old steamed veggies: lemon juice is an old favourite; curry powder (especially home-made) can really add punch; a vinaigrette can also work well;

reduced fat pestos will liven up an otherwise plain dish. For more ideas, see the recipes at the end of chapter 8.

STARCH STEALER

'What I say is that, if a man really likes potatoes, he must be a pretty decent sort of fellow.'

— A. A. MILNE

'Everything you see I owe to spaghetti.'

— SOPHIA LOREN

If you have a score greater than 40 on the Starches section of the questionnaire, chances are you are a Starch Stealer. Welcome to the club. It's a very big club indeed. Most of the people in the world get most of their calories from these types of foods. Even though we are berated for eating so much fat, it is still starchy carbohydrates that dominate our diets.

These starchy carbs are the newest nutritional battleground. There are entire sections of diet books dedicated to 'carbohydrate addicts' and their 'carbohydrate cravings'. And I know these cravings are real: I have patients who tell me they dream about bread and potatoes and rice when they are on a diet that forbids these foods. Despite the clamorous confusion and our limited (though rapidly growing) knowledge, let's try to make sense of it.

Starches: The Good News

When doctors and nutritionists advocate a way of eating that they believe will promote health and weight loss for most people, they usually recommend a low-fat, high-carbohydrate diet. What they are suggesting is that we should get fewer of our calories from fats and meats and more of our calories from pasta, rice, bread and potatoes as well as fruits and vegetables. If you look at the food pyramid on page 126, you will see that at the bottom of the graphic, the food group we should eat the most of is breads and other starches. Those recommendations were based on strong epidemio-logical evidence that this way of eating is associated with a lower risk of obesity and heart disease.

Many of these foods are low in calories and high in nutrition. They are also high in bulk. They take up a substantial amount of room in your stomach so you can fill up without consuming too many calories, and that's important.

Starches and other carbohydrates are also easily converted to glucose, the preferred body fuel. When you eat these foods, you are providing the energy your brain and body need in the form they like the best. And that's good.

Finally, research has shown that many people prefer eating high-carbohydrate foods – especially sweets – when they are stressed. In a study done in London, researchers recruited 68 healthy men and women to participate in an investigation of 'the effects of hunger on physiology, performance and mood'. Half were told that they would be expected to give a 4-minute speech after lunch and were given 10 minutes to prepare a talk on an assigned topic. The other half was instructed to listen to a tape on which a man read poetry by Dylan Thomas. After 10 minutes at each activity, the group was reunited and served lunch. Blood pressure, heart rate and mood were assessed for each person before and after the 10-minute activity. It's important to point out that not everyone in the speech group felt stressed by the task. Stress isn't just what happens, but how we respond to it.

At lunch, there were a variety of foods available from which each participant was free to choose. The amount each person ate during the first 15 minutes of the meal was carefully measured. Those who were stressed by their speech-preparation task ate a higher propor-tion of sweets and fats and consumed more calories than those who

WHY STRESS MAKES YOU CRAVE CARBS

Researchers at the Massachusetts Institute of Technology (MIT) in the 1970s found that carbohydrate consumption by rats promoted the production of serotonin in their brains. This is how it works: carbs increase insulin; insulin makes cells take up glucose and most amino acids (the most basic component of proteins). One amino acid that is not taken up by cells when insulin is around is tryptophan. Instead, tryptophan is taken up in the brain. This uptake is normally blocked by the presence of other amino acids, so having low levels of them in the blood makes it possible for tryptophan to better enter the brain, where it is converted to serotonin, an important mood stabilizer. This process initially described in rats has since been witnessed in people.

Researchers set up a live-in facility at MIT and invited overweight men and women to stay there while they studied them. What they ate was carefully monitored in their own special cafeteria, and they were able to snack as they wanted using specially designed vending machines. They were given a 'credit' card that allowed them to choose whatever they desired from the machines: fruit, sweets, biscuits, crisps, yoghurt – you name it.

After a couple of weeks, the researchers looked at what the live-in subjects had eaten, and an interesting pattern emerged. Many of them would eat normally at mealtimes, but then take in almost as many calories with snacks from the vending machines. Most of these snacks were high-carbohydrate foods. Moreover, these people did not eat snacks all day long, but tended to eat the same kind of foods at the same time each day. Later interviews with the subjects showed that the stimulus for the snack was a mood change and that eating the snack reversed the mood. The researchers concluded that these people were using the carbohydrates as a drug to treat their bad feelings.

didn't feel stressed. Why did the stress generated by the anxiety about giving a speech cause the subjects to choose starchy (and fat-laden) foods?

Research suggests that for some people, eating carbohydrates can actually stabilize their moods by changing the chemicals in their brains. For these people, starchy carbs are an instant antidote for stress. They should be on a low-fat, high-carb diet so they can incorporate their needed carbohydrates into their daily meals and snacks.

Starches: The Bad News

One of the problems with starches is that they are very easy to overeat. They are often warm and somewhat bland in taste, and they just feel good going down. Because of this, I recommend that you try serving yourself modest portions of these yummy foods initially. If you are still hungry, you can go back for more. Basically, I want you to *un*-supersize it and see what it really takes to make you feel full. For instance, a serving of pasta is 60g (2oz). A serving of rice is 75g (2½oz), and a serving of potatoes is one medium-size potato.

Finally, when you are preparing your starchy meal or snack, keep energy density in mind. You can eat 60g (2oz) of pasta with a little red sauce, and that might make you feel full, or you could spice it up with some very low density foods – mushrooms, green peppers and squash steamed or sautéed in a tiny amount of olive oil. That combination will increase the amount of food you eat without increasing the number of calories much. It allows you to have your starch and eat it too. And (need I even say this?) when you are eating a naturally low-density starch, don't make it denser by deep-fat frying it or covering it with fat; make it *less* dense by adding fibre or vegetables to it so that a little carbohydrate can really take you a long way.

Tips for Starch Stealers, No Matter What Diet You Are On

1. Choose low-glycaemic-load starches over those with a high glycaemic load. For a list of foods and their glycaemic loads, see page 129.

2. When your starch craving comes from stress, think about other ways you can manage your stress. Trying to deal with the cause of stress may be the best way to get rid of your craving. Take a walk and think about why you really need that doughnut or biscuit. Taking a short break often gets rid of the craving as well as the stress.

3. When you have a starch as part of a meal, serve yourself a modest portion and go back for seconds if you are still hungry.

For carbohydrate counters: I can only recommend starches as a very occasional treat. One of the ways this diet works is by limiting the foods you can eat and in that way limiting the calories you take in. On the other hand, if you crave an occasional starch, who am I to criticize? Just consider them the once-in-a-while treats, rather than daily fare. If your supermarket doesn't carry low-carb items, plenty of websites are dying to sell them to you, like the ones listed below. Order with caution. You don't want to eat them often.

www.LowCarbInternational.co.uk

www.LowCarbMegastore.co.uk

www.sugarfreesuperstore.co.uk

www.ukdiet.net

For calorie counters: With this type of food, portion control is tough. One trick that works for some of my patients is to eat the starch at the end of the meal, not at the beginning. Start with the protein-containing food and the vegetable, and then finish with the starch. It's much easier not to overeat when you are almost full.

For fat counters: Many starches come attached to fats, often saturated fats. This is particularly true of sweet starches and baked goods like cakes, muffins, pastries, biscuits or bagels. The fat can give these foods a low glycaemic load but still add on the calories. And calories *always* count. Try to find substitutes for your favourite high-fat starches that will limit your calorie intake. You can try buying a smaller one of whatever it is, or try new and lower-calorie foods and see if that helps.

SWEETS EATER

'Chocolate is a perfect food, as wholesome as it is delicious, a beneficent restorer of exhausted power. It is the best friend of those engaged in literary pursuits.'
    – BARON JUSTUS VON LIEBIG, FOUNDER OF AGRICULTURAL CHEMISTRY

'All I really need is love, but a little chocolate now and then doesn't hurt!'
    – LUCY VAN PELT (IN *PEANUTS*, BY CHARLES M. SCHULZ)

If you have a score higher than 40 on the Sweets portion of the questionnaire, then chances are you are a Sweets Eater. Actually, we all start off in life as Sweets Eaters; research has shown that infants instinctively prefer sweet tastes above all other tastes, and breast milk is perfectly designed to meet that demand. As a child grows, this preference decreases, but how much is variable. (Even in young children, you can see that some prefer sweets while others prefer more salty or savoury treats. I call it the sweets-versus-crisps difference.)

While many people who struggle with their weight regret their love of sweets, I think that like anything you really love, the job is to figure out how to integrate it into a way of eating that works for you and your own taste preference.

Sweets: The Good News

The love of sweets is certainly built-in at a very basic level. Anything that is this innate can't be all bad. In fact, a study published a few years ago suggested that moderate confectionery consumption, like moderate wine consumption, can prolong your life. People who eat one to three pieces of confectionery a month – I did say *moderate* consumption – can add an average of 1 year to their lives.

Why do we love sweets? There is good evidence that consumption of these foods can stimulate the opiate receptors – one of the primary pleasure sites we have in our brains. Researchers studying mice noted that eating sweets affected the same part of the rodents' brains that was affected by narcotics. Similar studies in humans have produced similar results.

Thus, there may be a physiologic foundation to the sense some people have that they are 'addicted' to sweets. In another series of studies, mice and rats were exposed to high levels of sweet foods. When they were cut off from their supply, their little paws trembled, and they were nervous and jumpy. Basically, the researchers reported, they were going through the rodent version of withdrawal. This doesn't mean that chocolate is the same as heroin. But I think it shows that our love for sweets is part of the way we are programmed at the genetic level and not some aberration.

If a love of sweets is hardwired into the brain, willpower alone will not be enough to make you resist these cravings. You have to outsmart them.

Sweets: The Bad News

When we look at whole populations, it becomes clear that a higher consumption of sweets is associated with higher weight. So, while fats might not make you fat, too many sweets probably will. When you separate fat consumption from sugar consumption, it's clear that a high-sweets diet is more likely to contribute to weight gain than a high-fat diet (though that's not always easy to do, since so many high-carbohydrate foods are also high-fat foods). Why is this, since sweets don't have any more calories than other foods? (In fact, sweets have only 4 calories per gram compared to fat, which has 9 calories a gram, or alcohol, which has 7 calories per gram.) There are probably two answers. First, I think it's clear that our bodies process sugary treats differently than other foods. No other food triggers our opiate receptors. Perhaps because of this, people who love sweets tend to overeat them in a way in which they might not be tempted to overeat other foods.

In addition, there is some evidence that suggests that leptin, the hormone that is produced by fat cells to protect your fat stores, affects how things taste. High leptin levels, which are found during times of weight maintenance, are associated with a decreased preference for sweets – at least in mice. Mice with low leptin levels (the way we humans are when we're losing weight) show a much stronger preference for sweet foods. If these findings are reproduced in humans, it will be just one more way that we are hardwired to love sweets and to use these foods to protect our precious fat stores.

From my perspective, a high-confectionery diet has another problem. A diet that's high in sweets is often low in fruits and vegetables. Whatever your perfect diet may be, in the long run, a diet that's high in fruits and vegetables is clearly the healthiest. Fruits and vegetables provide essential disease-fighting and cancer-preventing nutrients, they provide fibre, and they should be in everyone's diet. Unfortunately, Sweets Eaters tend to avoid fruits and vegetables.

Nevertheless, I am convinced that there is a way to incorporate sweets into your diet that allows you to eat a good diet and control your weight.

Sweets: The Plan

How you want to deal with your sweet cravings depends on how you crave them. Some people must have them every day; others want them only at times of stress; up to half of women who crave sweets do so on the days before their periods. I notice that I crave sweets only after I have had them. That is, if I eat a piece of confectionery, I want one the next day. If I don't eat any for a couple of days, I won't crave it. Probably many other patterns exist too.

There is evidence that sweets can be incorporated into a healthy diet without wreaking havoc on weight control. In Montreal, researchers took a group of people with diabetes – the very people who are usually taught to avoid sugary sweets at all costs – and randomly divided them into two groups. One group got the usual nutritional advice; the people in the other group were taught to allow 10 per cent of their daily calories to come from sugary treats. After 6 months, the sweets eaters ate fewer calories and gained less weight than the group who got the usual teaching.

So it can be done. But you have learn to plan around your sweets eating the same way you plan around all your other dietary goals. If you don't, and just hope for the best, then when you do succumb to your cravings (which is almost inevitable), you will be adding sweet treats on top of your full diet, and that inevitably causes weight gain.

I find that most of my patients do best when they include sweet foods in most of their meals. At breakfast, you might try peanut butter on your toast. Eat fruits at snack times and plan on having a dessert after lunch or dinner. In all my meal plans, I have included some sweets every day. The exception is the 30-gram Counting Carbohydrates Diet, where the carbohydrate limit is too low to include more than a single sweet on most days.

Try to have the sweet when you are at home, where you have

arranged choices that you can feel good about. Try not to eat desserts when you eat out. Restaurant servings of sweets, like all their servings of foods, are much too large. For most people, providing sweets as part of a scheduled meal or snack reduces cravings at other times.

However, those extracurricular cravings will still come to most Sweets Eaters. When do you have most of your cravings? Most Sweets Eaters have cravings in the afternoon or evening. Researchers at MIT have also shown that many Sweets Eaters and other carb cravers tend to get their cravings at the same, predictable times each day.

This is where your food diary will come in very handy. Find out when you are most likely to crave sweets and then figure out how to satisfy your urge in a way that allows you to feel good about yourself and your weight.

When you get a craving for sweets, take a minute to think about where it's coming from. Are you stressed? Depressed? Lonely? Angry? These are common reasons I hear from my patients. Consider trying some other way to deal with your craving. Exercise is an excellent way to cope with many of these feelings. See if you can take a walk, a bike ride, an exercise class. If you still have the craving after the exercise, by all means eat a treat – at least you will have burned some extra calories.

One of the patients I've told you about, Diane, came to my office not long ago, glowing with triumph. She had been tormented by cravings for sweets late at night, right before bed. She tried fruit, gum, even sugar-free sweets. Nothing worked except chocolate. Still, she didn't like eating the chocolate right before bed. I had encouraged her to try exercise, and that hadn't worked either. She recognized that the craving came from a bad feeling she was having, but she couldn't figure out what she really wanted. Finally, it occurred to her that maybe she was lonely. The kids were in bed, the news on TV was all bad, she was tired, but this feeling, this longing for company kept her from going to bed. So instead of eating chocolate, she started calling her sister, also her best friend, when she felt this hunger at night. It worked, and she hadn't eaten a snack at night in more than 3 weeks. She felt empowered. She felt good.

When you get the craving for sweets, choose a sweet you can eat and still face yourself in the mirror later. Of course, that means not overeating. So, no matter which diet you are on, choose a sweet that's low in calories. If you are on a fat-counting diet, choose one that is low in fats. If you are on a carbohydrate-counting diet, you're going to have a hard time getting any variety into your sweet treats, because most sweets are carbohydrates. Still, it can be done, and I have some tips below just for you.

You might think that a taste of what you crave is not going to be enough. You will be surprised. Sweets cravings, like many food cravings, are mediated through your mouth and its taste equipment. Your mouth has no ability to quantify how much you are eating. It only knows *whether* you are eating or not, so when you choose to give yourself the treat of your dreams, you can probably get away with really satisfying that craving with a much smaller serving than you are used to.

My sister Shelley loves McDonald's McFlurries. There have been times in her life when she had to have one every day. But she discovered that she could order a small one and it was just as satisfying as a large. And more recently, there are even days when she can take a few spoonfuls and then throw the rest out, because she's satisfied.

Sweets may be the hardest food to incorporate into a rational diet, but if you are a Sweets Eater, it's important to take on that challenge. After all, it's unlikely that your preference will change, so you have to figure out a way to live with it if you want to manage your weight. The world we live in makes just saying no an unrealistic plan for those of us who have a love affair with sweets.

I've included a list of a few of the millions of sweet treats you might consider. Here are the qualities I look for in a treat.

- The treat should be low in calories.

- It can be purchased in small snack-size amounts.

- It comes in a form that allows you to easily understand and consume only the amount you want – for example, calorie counts that allow the snack to be divided into easily understood quantities, for example, the whole bar or this many pieces.

LOW-CALORIE SWEETS

Sweet Treat	Calories	Fat (g)	Carbohydrate (g)
After-dinner mint, 1 (6g)	87	1.5	11
Boiled sweets, 5	100	0	25
Butterscotch, 4	96	0	22
Chewing gum (most brands) 1 piece	10	0	2
Chocolate caramel, 1 (20g)	99	5.5	12
Chocolate-coated whipped bar 1 (26g)	103	4.1	16.5
Fresh fruit salad, 145g (5oz)	77	0.1	19.3
Frozen yoghurt, light 170g (6oz)	120	2	20
Fruit gums 60g (2oz)	16	0	54
Ice cream (vanilla, light), 100ml	83	6	12
Jelly babies, 5	8	0	2
Jelly beans, 10	100	0	26
Maltesers (½ packet)	106	4.25	15
Peppermints, 1 packet	84	0	0
Raspberry lolly, 1 (90ml)	107	3.5	17.5
Toffees, 5	100	2.5	17.5

- It's something that you like, but not something you need to binge on; if you know you can't eat chocolate in moderation, don't buy chocolate.

Tips for Sweets Eaters, No Matter What Diet You Are On

1. Clear the house of everything you don't want to eat. Don't just keep stuff stashed away. Throw it out.

2. Always have something sweet at hand that you will feel good about eating. You can try having fruit around; very sweet fruits like grapes and melon can work for some people, at least part of the time. Frozen fruit bars might work. Low-calorie ice cream bars sometimes do the trick.

3. Have a variety of healthy sweet treats around the house and only one type of sweet that you could crave but wouldn't want to eat too much of. That will improve your odds of satisfying your craving with a food that you won't be sorry you ate.

4. Only have as much of the restricted sweet in the house as you would want to eat at any given moment. Buy serving sizes and, if necessary, buy them one at a time. Then replace your stock when you are not having cravings, so that you will be prepared next time they come.

5. Have a plan for what to do when the wholesome sweets at hand don't do it for you. The nature of that plan will depend on you and your cravings. Janet (remember her?) has a real sweet tooth and loves ice cream. When she craves ice cream and nothing else will do, she makes herself walk to get it. She lives in a large city, and there is a local store nearby. She figures the walk (and the hassle) into her craving calculations.

6. If you feel that you can never learn to eat sweets in moderation and decide that the only way you can deal with your 'addiction' is to ban sweets forever, have a plan for what to do if you 'fall off the wagon'. Having no plan means leaving your diet in the hands of chance and whim. My whole point is that you do better in managing what you eat if you have a plan and choose what to eat, no matter how hard that is. You need to take charge of your diet, and that means staying in charge even when you can't control all your cravings all the time.

7. Finally, anticipate how you will feel after you've eaten something you hadn't planned on. Too often the response is 'I'll start again tomorrow', and that can trigger a binge. Be proactive in the face of what might feel like a failure. When you are late paying a bill, you don't say, 'Oh well, I'll pay that bill next month'. Same with unintended splurges. Try to get back on track, that day, that hour, that very minute – and go from there.

For carbohydrate counters: If you love sweets, then a carbohydrate-counting diet is going to be pretty darn tough. These foods need to be eaten in moderation, especially when you are in the early phase of the diet and want to stay 'in the pink'. Have only a small amount of sweet foods to hand. Make sure these foods are the ones you can eat without regret.

Here are some foods you can eat in moderation, even in the early phase.

- Strawberries, blueberries and raspberries
- Sugarless confectionery or gum (These snacks have a built-in overeating prevention mechanism: they can give you powerful and very regrettable gas when eaten in excess.)
- A small swirl of Anchor Light aerosol cream or even a dab of real whipped cream to brighten up fruits

Remember, although sugarless items don't have carbohydrates, they do contain calories. Moderation in all things is key.

For calorie counters: Portion control is key in eating sweets, so give yourself an edge.

- Only have as much in the house as you would want to eat at any given moment.
- Have a variety of healthy sweet treats around and only one type of sweet that you could crave but wouldn't want to eat often. The greater the variety of sweets around you, the greater the quantity of sweets you tend to eat. Use that understanding to try to ease your craving with a variety of wholesome, low-calorie treats.

For fat counters: Avoid chocolate. It is loaded with fats and, in general, the higher the quality of chocolate, the greater the amount of fat, most of it saturated. Here are some good rules of thumb for all sweets.

- Check out the fat content of all the sweets you eat – biscuits, pastries and other baked goods are usually dripping with fats. Find out how much fat is in a sweet, and if it contains more than 33 per cent fat, choose again.
- Avoid low-fat versions of sweets if you can. The fat is usually replaced with sugar, and sugar can make you fat too.

WATERLESS WONDER

'Some say the glass is half empty, some say the glass is half full; I say, are you going to drink that?'

— LISA CLAYMEN

If you had a score of 30 or less, there is a good chance you're not drinking enough.

When I first started keeping my own diet diary, I was shocked to see that on most days I drank only coffee with perhaps a glass of wine at the end of the day. Others have reported the same pattern.

The usual recommendation is that everyone should drink eight 220ml (8fl oz) glasses of water each day. Most books on nutrition will recommend this. What's the science here? Well, there isn't a lot.

So what should a rational person do? Let's start with the basics: water is an essential nutrient. And we have only limited capabilities to store water. While our bodies are 70 per cent water, that water is being used and is necessary. Moreover, we lose water every day. If we count only the water we lose by breathing and sweating – without even exercising – we lose 2 to 4 litres of water per day. That's not including urine or stools. Without water, the average person will die in 2 to 5 days, well before she would die from lack of food. So, water is important in the diet, in some ways even more important than food.

What is the optimal amount of water to drink when you are losing weight? Many diet books will tell you that drinking water helps flush fat and promotes weight loss. Maybe. There isn't any scientific literature on this, and you should know that anecdotal evidence – such as, 'It worked for my Aunt Minnie' – is wrong at least as often as it is right.

When there is no data, opinion can flourish, so I'll give you my opinion. I think drinking a lot of water is good for you. I think it makes you feel better. I think it makes you look better and that your skin actually looks younger when you are well-hydrated. And I think water consumption can contribute to weight loss. I'm not convinced that it helps 'flush out' fat, except in the same sense that water flushes out much of our waste products.

I suspect that water consumption promotes weight loss, first, by contributing to our satiety (volume in the stomach helps to make you feel full) and, second, by helping us feel healthier. When we are clinically dehydrated, our bodies don't work well; physical performance can suffer when we lose as little as 455 to 900g (1 to 2lb) of water, and mental performance is measurably decreased when we lose 3.6 to 4.5kg (8 to 10lb) of water. And mild to moderate dehydration has been linked to increased risk of bladder cancer (very rare in this country) and colon cancer (not so rare here).

So I say, drink up. Here's how you can tell if you are drinking enough water: your urine should be very pale in colour. If it's yellow or tan-coloured, you aren't getting enough water.

If your heart is sinking at the prospect of drinking that much water, cheer up. Other fluids can provide the water you need plus some flavouring. Milk counts as a fluid; so do soft drinks. Juice counts as well. Even if you count those other drinks, chances are that you still fall short of your goal of eight glasses a day. How can you get all that water in?

I try to drink two glasses of water every morning even before my coffee. Now I have a good start on my goal. And I try to drink one glass of water with every meal and snack. I frequently substitute either a soft drink or tea for water, especially with my snacks, but I have to admit that I have developed a real love for plain cold water, especially first thing in the morning. I also drink at least one glass of low-fat milk in my coffee over the course of a day, and on a good day that gets me to my target of eight glasses a day.

If you are exercising, you're going to need even more fluid. Every year we get a news story about a young, extremely fit marine or football player who doesn't drink enough water. He or she gets overheated from too much exertion and gets carried off the field on a stretcher. If he's lucky, he survives. When you exercise, especially when it's hot but other times as well, drink *before* you play, drink *as* you play, and drink *after* you play. Your performance will be improved, and you will feel better.

Not everything that is served in a glass will count towards the magic goal of eight glasses per day. Following are brief descriptions of what we know about some of the different types of drinks in a normal British diet. 'Beverage Pros and Cons' on page 276 summarizes these findings.

What about Coffee?

'The morning cup of coffee has an exhilaration about it which the cheering influence of the afternoon or evening cup of tea cannot be expected to reproduce.'
— OLIVER WENDELL HOLMES, SR., AUTHOR

That exhilaration comes at least in part from the caffeine in the coffee, and caffeine is a mild diuretic. (A diuretic is a drug that promotes water loss.) So, you can't count on coffee to replace the water you lose.

Perhaps because of the caffeine and the exhilaration it produces, there is a sense that coffee is somehow bad for you and that tea is somehow good for you. This is a very old belief; researchers have been trying to pin down the truth for hundreds of years. The earliest controlled trial I have come across was actually conducted in 18th-century Sweden. A pair of identical twins had been sentenced to death for murder. King Gustave III thought that rather than execute these twins, he would put them to work in service to science. He spared the gallows-bound twins in return for their participation in a controlled trial of coffee drinking versus tea drinking. One twin had to drink three large bowls of tea every day, and his brother had to drink the same amount of coffee. Both outlived the curious king. But the tea drinker died first, at the ripe old age of 83. His coffee-consuming brother joined him in the graveyard just a couple of months later. I'm not sure that counts as a coffee victory.

But science has continued to consider this question. Here's what we know: coffee increases blood pressure in those who drink it occasionally, although this doesn't appear to happen in habitual coffee drinkers. Coffee has been linked to elevated LDL cholesterol and other components that increase heart disease, but there is no evidence that coffee itself increases heart disease, despite many studies.

Researchers have tried, without much success, I must add, to link coffee to all kinds of awful health outcomes in addition to heart disease: miscarriages and cancer, mostly. So far none of these connections have been confirmed. It's thought that much of the apparent guilt of coffee is by association – due to lifestyle factors that often accompany coffee drinking, such as smoking. So, for now, coffee has a pretty clean bill of health.

Bottom line: drink coffee if you enjoy it, but don't count it as a beverage when you are trying to determine whether or not you are getting enough to drink.

How about Tea?

'If you are cold, tea will warm you – if you are too heated, it will cool you – if you are depressed, it will cheer you – if you are excited, it will calm you.'
    – WILLIAM GLADSTONE

Tea has always had a patina of virtue about it, kind of the flip side to the dark aura of coffee. As it turns out, tea is full of antioxidants known as polyphenols and, at least in the laboratory, these ingredients have been shown to have effects that would reduce risk of heart disease and cancer in humans. Does it pan out in reality? It's not clear. Some studies have shown benefits to tea drinking; others have not. Tea drinking, like coffee drinking, has associated lifestyle factors that make measuring its effects more difficult.

By the way, when the virtues of tea are discussed, they are associated only with black tea, green tea or oolong tea. All of these come from the leaves of the *Camellia sinensis*. The other types of infusions, which are usually called herbal teas, don't really count as teas. And while they count towards your daily intake of liquids they don't contain polyphenols.

I'm from the American South, where you always have two tea choices, both iced: sweet tea or plain. And when they say sweet, they mean it. When you drink that sweet tea, Southern style, it might as well be a cola. That's okay in small quantities, but adding sugar to tea just increases its calories.

Bottom line: drink tea if you enjoy it; it may even be good for you. Just don't load it up with sugar.

What about Juice?

Let me reveal a prejudice here: I don't get juice drinking. I like the occasional V-8 juice and some homemade juices, but from my perspective, juice has lots of calories, little or no fibre and a reduced amount of vitamins. If you ate the fruit itself rather than drinking the juice, you would get fewer calories, more fibre and more vitamins. Plus you would feel fuller.

Can you have a glass of juice every now and then because you like it? Sure, but don't drink it because you think it's really good for you. Yes there are some good packaged juices out there but watch out for those with added sugar. And always remember that they add a lot of calories without filling you up.

Bottom line: drink juices sparingly; if you love the taste, use a touch of them to flavour your water.

How about Soft Drinks?

Obviously, soft drinks contain lots and lots of sugar. And lately they come in 500ml bottles and cups that you can practically bathe in, so it's very easy to overconsume them.

Here's something else about soft drinks: they can make you fat – and not just because they're loaded with calories. There is something else going on here. Over the past 20 years, soft drink manufacturers (and manufacturers of other sweet products as well) have stopped using cane sugar – you know, the white stuff that comes in a bag at the supermarket. They have replaced cane sugar with a sweetener made from corn. Corn sweeteners contain a type of sugar called fructose. In your body, fructose acts differently than glucose – the sugar most commonly found in your system. For example, glucose requires insulin in order to be taken up into cells. Fructose doesn't. Fructose also reduces circulating leptin levels. Both insulin and leptin play important roles in getting us to quit eating at the end of a meal or snack, so there is some concern that fructose is helping us get fat by allowing us to take in calories without feeling their filling effect. (It just goes to show you how complicated our bodies are – too much insulin can make you fat; it turns out that too little may also.)

Fructose consumption in test animals induces insulin resistance, impaired glucose tolerance, high blood pressure and high triglyceride levels. The data in humans are less clear, although there is some evidence that it can affect us the same way it does mice. From my perspective, this is yet another reason to avoid soft drinks.

Bottom line: if you like soft drinks, you can drink them on occasion. If you can tolerate the switch to diet, drink that. If not, then think of a soft drink as a treat, like dessert, to be indulged in rarely and savoured fully.

What about Alcohol?

'Burgundy makes you think of silly things; Bordeaux makes you talk about them; and Champagne makes you do them.'
    – JEAN ANTHELME BRILLAT-SAVARIN

Alcohols contain 7 calories per gram, almost twice what soft drinks have. So when you drink, you are loading up on calories. On the other hand, we rarely drink alcohol, with the possible exception of beer, in the sort of quantities that characterize how many of us drink soft drinks.

The other problem with alcohol is – well, your mother was right – it lowers your inhibitions. It lowers your inhibitions about drinking more; it also lowers your inhibitions about eating more. Research has shown that drinking wine with meals causes people to stay longer at the table and to consume more food calories. A glass of wine with dinner is a pleasure, but just assume that when you drink with a meal, you will also eat more.

In addition, alcohol has some diuretic effects. One of the reasons (although not the only one) you feel so bad the day after you drink too much is that you are dehydrated. Drinking alcohol causes a net fluid loss, so it doesn't count towards your eight glasses a day.

On the other hand, alcohol has been shown to decrease the risk of heart disease. In a study of 38,000 American male doctors and dentists, men who drank moderately (between one and three glasses, five to seven nights a week) had a lower risk of heart disease than those who didn't drink at all. And – this is surprising – it didn't seem to matter whether they drank beer or wine.

Bottom line: avoid alcohol when you are actively trying to lose weight; when your weight is stable, alcohol in moderation can improve your health. And because it's a diuretic, it doesn't count towards your eight-glass goal.

Tips for Waterless Wonders, No Matter What Diet You Are On

For carbohydrate counters: Drinking your basic eight glasses of water a day is particularly important for you for two reasons. First, a diet low in carbs is high in proteins. No matter what you eat, you have to drink enough water to flush the waste out, and with proteins there is more waste. In order to deal with this, you will need to drink extra water. The second reason is that constipation is a big complaint of many on this diet – at least in the early part. Water can help prevent constipation. Eight glasses will be enough; make sure you get that much water every day.

BEVERAGE PROS AND CONS

Drink	Pros	Cons	Bottom Line
Alcohol	Modest alcohol consumption improves cardiovascular risk factors	Contains 7 calories per gram; lowers inhibitions, which promotes overeating	Avoid alcohol while actively trying to lose weight. Limit alcohol intake to 1 (women) or 2 (men) drinks per night to maximize benefits and reduce risks. Does not count towards your 8 glasses.
Coffee	A good medium for milk	Caffeine is a diuretic	Caffeinated coffee doesn't count towards your 8 glasses.
Herbal tea	Has no caffeine	Often gets loaded with sugar	Counts towards your 8 glasses.
Milk	Dairy products promote bone growth and weight loss	Contains lots of saturated fats and carbohydrates	Drink skimmed or semi-skimmed milk to reduce the amount fat in your diet. Counts towards your 8 glasses.
Tea	Has antioxidants in it; has much less caffeine than in coffee	Often gets loaded with sugar	Counts towards your 8 glasses.
Soft drinks	Contain lots of water	Contain lots of sugar; may promote weight gain	Counts towards your 8 glasses. Drink diet soft drinks to reduce overall calorie intake.

For calorie counters: You will be taking in more protein as you cut calories, so make sure you get enough water to flush out the waste products left over after you use the proteins. Watch your urine, and if it looks darker than water, you need to drink more liquids.

For fat counters: You will be eating foods that have a very high water content, so your need for extra liquid is lower than those on the other types of diets. Still, you need to monitor your urine. If it looks darker than water, increase the amount of water you drink.

PROP TASTER

'An onion can make people cry, but there has never been a vegetable invented to make them laugh.'

— WILL ROGERS (A SUSPECTED PROP TASTER)

If you scored 40 or higher on the PROP Test, chances are that you are what is known as a taster, and if you scored higher than 80, you may even be a supertaster. PROP is a naturally occurring chemical in food that's only real importance is the bitterness of its taste. If you can taste it, you are genetically programmed to dislike important and health-promoting foods such as broccoli, spinach, Brussels sprouts, cabbage and grapefruit. As it turns out, liking these vegetables and fruits may be the odd quality, since up to 75 per cent of the world's population are tasters and a mere 25 per cent non-tasters, that is, people who are insensitive to the bitterness of many of the foods that are so good for you.

When researchers have studied tasters and supertasters, they have found that, in general, both groups dislike Brussels sprouts, cauliflower, cabbage, radishes and grapefruit more than non-tasters. Other foods disliked by tasters include coffee, green tea and bitter beers. In addition, the group described as supertasters tend to dislike foods that are very sweet or that have a high fat content. This makes supertasters perhaps the pickiest eaters in the world.

Is there an association between your PROP-taster status and weight? It makes sense, but so far the studies are not conclusive. In some surveys, supertasters were thinner than non-tasters. Why would they be thinner? Since supertasters have many more food aversions than non-tasters, it is possible that they eat a very bland, unvaried diet, and diets with less variety have been associated with a lower BMI.

If how things taste is determined by your genes, you can't be blamed for not eating your broccoli. Doctors and nutritionists have insisted that we all should eat a diet low in fat and high in fruits and vegetables. The fact that these foods don't taste good to a significant portion of the population hasn't really even been discussed.

The genetic basis of taste is not a new discovery. In the 1930s, a chemist named A. L. Fox was working with a chemical very similar to PROP, and some of it accidentally became airborne. Fox's colleague immediately noted and commented on the bitter taste of the airborne stuff, but Fox himself tasted nothing. That simple observation led to hundreds of family studies investigating the genetic varieties in the ability to taste PROP.

Since then, populations across the globe have been tested for this trait. In Western Africa, 97 per cent of the population are tasters. In India, only 60 per cent are. In the adult populations of the US and UK, 75 per cent are tasters. In general, the ability to taste PROP is strongest when you are younger and declines slowly with age. It's more common in women than men. In women, the ability to taste PROP is influenced by sex hormones, so it fluctuates over the course of the menstrual cycle and in pregnancy.

Although exactly how this trait works is not well understood, there are measurable differences between tasters, non-tasters and supertasters. For one thing, tasters have more tastebuds than non-tasters, and supertasters have even more than tasters. And some researchers have found that there are different sensitivities to different types of bitterness even among tasters – that some of us may be more sensitive to the taste of quinine; others, to the taste of PROP. Current thinking is that there may be up to 60 different receptors just for the perception of bitterness.

This is an active area of research, simply because what we eat is important and many of the foods currently thought of as good for us (such as fruits and vegetables) are not widely consumed despite active encouragement. The reason doctors and nutritionists want you to eat these fruits and vegetables is that they contain disease-reducing chemicals that can help you stay healthy longer. In a number of population-based studies like the Harvard Nurses' Study, higher consumption of fruits and vegetables was associated with lower rates of many cancers as well as lower rates of obesity and heart disease.

The goal of this research is to see if there is a biological and genetic reason for our eating habits and then try to fix it. So, if you hate broccoli, as does the former US president, George Bush *père*, consider that this may be inherited. You can't help it if you don't like it; you got it from your mum or dad. On the other hand, research also indicates that sensitivity to bitterness is highest in young children, and this is the age when food preferences are determined. It is possible that the vegetable you hated as a child tastes pretty good now – but first you have to taste it.

The other thing to do, since fruits and vegetables are an important part of a diet and grossly underconsumed, is to actively look for ones you like. Too often, we are introduced to only a few vegetables before our mothers throw up their hands in despair and give up. We generalize from our experience with broccoli and spinach that we do not like vegetables. Let me encourage you to try other (non-bitter) vegetables and fruits. (A list of non-bitter fruits and vegetables is provided on page 280.) We live in a world where we can eat just about everything. Use this ability to expand your horizons vegetable-wise.

NON-BITTER VEGETABLES FOR PROP TASTERS

(The foods in **bold print** are best for the 30-gram Counting Carbohydrates Diet; all are acceptable on the 100-gram Counting Carbohydrates Diet.)

1. **Artichoke**
2. **Asparagus**
3. Aubergine
4. **Avocado**
5. Beans – virtually all varieties
6. Beetroot
7. Carrots
8. **Celery**
9. Chickpeas
10. **Cucumbers**
11. Green peppers
12. **Hot Peppers**
13. Jicama
14. **Leeks**
15. Lentils
16. **Lettuce (many varieties)**
17. **Mushrooms**
18. Okra
19. **Olives**
20. Parsnips
21. Peas
22. Potatoes
23. Pumpkin
24. **Soya beans, green**
25. Squash
26. Sweet potatoes
27. Sweetcorn
28. **Tomatoes**
29. Turnips
30. Yams

Tips for PROP Tasters, No Matter What Diet You Are On

1. Eat the youngest leaves of leafy greens. Often young leaves have much less of the bitter flavour than more mature leaves.

2. Cook bitter vegetables in ways that reduce their bitter flavours. The most common way is to cook the vegetable at a high heat

in a little olive oil with garlic. To enforce the fat-counting theme, use 1 to 2 tablespoons of olive oil and 60 to 120ml (2 to 4fl oz) fat-free chicken stock or white wine. Simmer until tender.

3. Salt decreases bitterness. Season bitter vegetables generously with salt and see if you like them more.

4. Combine vegetables with starches. It's one way to use the tang of the vegetables to liven up the smooth blandness of the starch.

5. Use small amounts of vegetables as ingredients in other dishes. This way you will increase your vegetable intake in an enjoyable way. Broccoli quiche is a classic example. There are others out there. Just look around.

6. Very few fruits have bitter flavours. Grapefruit is probably the worst. There are also rhubarb and persimmons. So if you can't get yourself past your loathing of vegetables, try to increase your intake of fruits from the wide variety nature offers.

For carbohydrate counters: One of the easiest ways to reduce the bitterness of many vegetables is to add salt and butter. While butter is nothing but saturated fat, and filled with calories, the benefit it offers in making these important foods palatable outweighs the downside, especially on this diet. So, as you are cooking, feel free to use a modest amount of butter to enhance the taste of vegetables, if that makes them more appealing.

You'll also find that many of these vegetables taste wonderful in a casserole made with eggs and cheese. Recipes for this type of casserole abound in cookbooks and on the Web.

For calorie counters: Most of these foods are wonderfully low in calories, so you can combine them with other foods to make them more palatable. Mixing greens or other bitter vegetables with a starch is a classic way of improving on both the tang of the vegetable and the blandness of the starch. Normally, bitter greens such as spinach and kale can be sautéed in oil and stock or wine and then added to a pasta for a different taste. Including these foods in your diet will increase your variety without increasing your calorie count, so try it; you'll like it.

For fat counters: Since fruits and vegetables will make up the bulk (literally) of what you eat, it's very important to expand your horizons if you are a PROP taster. In addition to trying new foods, try new ways of preparing the same old stuff. Asian cuisines – Indian, Thai, Chinese, Japanese – offer a variety of ways to cook these foods to minimize the bitterness that may be there. If you like them, you should invest in one or two good cookbooks to give you more ways to prepare these essential foods. A touch of exotic oil like walnut oil or sesame oil can bring new life and flavours to the same old dishes, and I encourage you to try some.

CHAPTER 10

DIETING HISTORY

VOLUME

'My doctor told me to stop having intimate dinners for four. Unless there are three other people.'

     — Orson Welles

If you selected mostly *a*'s in the What Makes You Feel Full section of the questionnaire, then one of your primary cues that you have eaten enough is volume. There are two aspects of volume: the first is visually determined and at least partially psychological. When you look at your plate, you think, 'This is (or is not) enough food to satisfy me.' Your assessment, which is based on how much it has previously taken to fill you, creates an expectation of satiety. The second aspect of volume is physiological: you eat a certain amount of food, and it fills you up – literally.

Let's talk about the visual cues first. One of the things I hear from my patients is that they sometimes have a sense when they are dieting that the amount of food they're eating simply isn't enough. They look at the recommended portion of meat – the size of their palm – and think, 'This can't possibly be enough to fill me up.' They know how much they normally eat, and that is not it.

It may have come as a surprise to you to hear that the judgement about what constitutes a normal-size portion is learned. It is based on how much you have eaten as a portion in the past. This learned response can change, and has changed a lot in recent decades. Over the past 25 years or so, thanks to the success of a guy named David Wallerstein, serving size has increased dramatically. Wallerstein (whose dubious achievement was recently described in the terrific book about the fattening of America, *Fat Land*, by Greg Critser) was trying to increase profits at a chain of movie theatres by getting theatregoers to buy more popcorn. But try as he might, he couldn't induce people to buy two bags. So he made larger single bags, and supersizing was born. It may not surprise you to hear that Wallerstein is now an executive at McDonald's.

Although supersizing is specific to fast-food places, the idea that you can make a lot more money by offering people a lot more food has permeated our society at every level. From chocolate bars to the foods served in our finest restaurants, portion size has gone up, up, up. Nouvelle cuisine was a phenomenon in the 1970s and 80s, and, although it was relatively popular, it tended to leave people with the feeling that they were not getting enough food for their money eating these beautiful but spare meals. As a result such meals now tend to be the preserve of very upmarket restaurants.

Marketers and researchers have demonstrated that portion size – that is, how much we think it will take to make us full – is learned and can change based on what is available. When presented with larger portions, people will eat up to 30 per cent more than they otherwise would. Human hunger is apparently quite elastic, which makes excellent evolutionary sense: our hunter-gatherer ancestors ate whenever the eating was good, thereby storing reserves of fat against future famine. The problem is that in an era of abundance, the opportunity for feasting now presents itself 24/7 – and at bargain prices.

Researchers in Sweden recruited 27 subjects, overweight and normal weight, and had them eat a meal on two separate occasions. Before each meal, they were asked how hungry they were, and after each meal, they were asked how satisfied they were. The first meal was a normal meal, and the second meal was eaten blindfolded. When blindfolded, the participants ate 20 per cent less of the same meal than they had when they could see the food. Seeing the food drove the participants to eat what they thought was their normal serving, even though less food would have been just as satisfying.

So, for those who have a strong visual component to their sense of fullness, know that it is adjustable in a way that other types of satiety are not.

The other kind of satisfaction provided by volume is the feeling that comes from your gastrointestinal tract. As researcher Barbara Rolls, PhD, demonstrated, many of us tend to eat the same volume of food, regardless of the calorie count. Here's how her research has been done. She recruits a group of volunteers – she's done these types of experiments on both normal-weight and overweight people – and she will feed these volunteers one or more meals in a given day. Then she asks them to write down everything they eat for the rest of that day. Each volunteer will do this several times over the course of the experiment. What the volunteers do not know is that, although the meals she prepares for them all look and taste similar, they have different amounts of calories: one meal might have a lot of calories; the next, many fewer. They eat and then record everything else they eat and drink for the next day or so after the meal. Typically, these studies last only a couple of days, but several have followed food amounts for up to 11 weeks.

Here's what Dr Rolls discovered: many people ate the same amount of food independent of the calories in the meal. That is, whether the meal was mostly pasta (lots of calories) or mostly veggies (many fewer calories), the volunteers ate the same volume of food in all the meals. And they didn't overeat later to compensate. Based on their food diaries, on days when the research meal was low in calories, they just ate fewer calories. Their level of hunger and satisfaction were the same. Thus researchers concluded that for many of us, volume is a more important aspect of satisfaction than calorie content.

If you're one of these people, you can fill yourself with low-calorie foods and feel just as full and satisfied as if you had eaten high-calorie foods. If so, you are most likely to do well on a low-fat diet that emphasizes the replacement of high-calorie fats with low-calorie carbohydrates.

Even within the category of carbohydrates, you can replace high-calorie carbs – pasta, rice, cakes and biscuits – with low-calorie substitutes like vegetables and fruits. You don't eliminate the pasta, but you replace some of it with a lower-calorie substitute, and you end up eating fewer calories but still feeling full.

Although those who depend on volume for satiety do well on the Counting Fats Diet, this principle will work with just about any other diet too.

Tips for Those Who Need Volume, No Matter What Diet They Are On

1. Use fruits and vegetables as the volume providers. Think of your plate as a pie chart; fill half of the plate with your fruits or vegetables, and the other half should be evenly divided between the meat and the starch.

2. Recalibrate your visual sense of what a serving is. To do this, measure all of your portions, at least for the first 2 weeks. Our expectations of what one serving is has crept up along with our weight.

3. Serve yourself food one portion at a time. Research has shown that the larger the serving, the more we eat; 115g (4oz) of meat may not seem like much, because our sense of portion is so out of whack, but it may fill you up. If it doesn't, you can always go back for seconds.

4. Don't buy economy-size anything. Studies have shown that the amount of food you expect to eat as a single portion increases as the size of the container it comes from increases.

For carbohydrate counters: The temptation for you is going to be to eat more protein and fat rather than carbohydrates in your search for more food. Don't do it. Serve yourself some more salad or vegetables and, if you are still hungry, consider seconds of the meat. If you really need volume to feel full, vegetables provide more bulk and volume than meat.

A rule of thumb: if you still feel hungry after you have eaten your meal, then you need more volume, so eat more vegetables. If you feel hungry again after an hour or two, then increase the size of your protein portion.

For calorie counters: Use high-calorie foods as flavourings for low-calorie foods. Your chilli should be more beans than meat; your stew should be more potatoes, carrots, onions and peas than meat. Strawberry shortcake should be heavy on the strawberries and light on the shortcake and whipped cream.

For fat counters: Combine starches with lower-calorie carbohydrates. When you make pasta or rice, add vegetables for flavour and volume.

VARIETY

'Variety is the soul of pleasure.'
    — APHRA BEHN

If you found yourself checking mostly *b*'s in the What Makes You Feel Full section, then you depend on eating enough variety to make you feel full and satisfied. The hardwired drive to crave a variety of foods makes itself felt at a very early age. Studies show that children as young as 3 years old will choose a diet composed of a variety of foods even if they've been offered a favourite food.

Researchers in England first noted in rhesus monkeys that the pleasure associated with any given food decreases as the food is eaten. And that was true even if the offered food was a favourite. After a relatively short while, the pleasure afforded by that food diminished enough so that the desire for other foods was stronger, and the monkeys stopped eating one food and started on another. The researcher named this phenomenon 'sensory-specific satiety'. As it turns out, humans work the same way. A food, no matter how loved, will lose some of its pleasure-giving power as soon as it is eaten so that other foods, even those less desirable, become more preferred. This is because variety offers us the best chance for obtaining all the nutrients essential in life.

If variety promotes eating more, then limiting variety ought to make it easier to eat less and easier to lose weight. This is certainly how many diets work. And it does work – for a while. But can you limit your food choices forever? I think some people can. We all know people who eat virtually the same foods day after day after day and seem to enjoy that. But for most of us, food choices are driven at least in part by a need for variety.

Many people have told me that one reason they found diets so hard to stick to is the limitation on the selection of foods. One of the greatest attributes of Weight Watchers is that, although it rewards a low-fat, low-calorie diet, *nothing* is forbidden. Variety is allowed, even encouraged. And Weight Watchers is at least as successful as other weight-loss programmes.

How is it possible for variety to promote obesity but also be used successfully in weight loss? Because the drive for variety resides in your mouth, and since this drive for any given food is quickly satisfied, and we, like the monkeys, can move on to the next food.

So, if you crave variety in your diet, then you can harness that to help you eat less food by eating a wider variety at each meal. But – and this is key – you must limit your portions so that you don't end up increasing your variety *and* the amount of food. If you can learn to enjoy a small portion of a wide variety of foods, this can be a successful strategy for losing weight. In fact, in my Counting Fats and Counting Calories Diets, I offer small portions of several foods at each meal to try to harness the power of variety and improve satisfaction despite limiting calories.

Tips for Those Who Need Variety, No Matter What Diet They Are On

1. Incorporate variety into all your meals. The temptation is to just eat a lot of a single food, particularly for the first two meals of the day – a bowl of cereal in the morning; the same green salad at lunch. Don't do it. It is more work, but you will find it easier to eat less overall if at every meal you include different food types and textures. Don't save that for dinner time when you are more likely to overeat.

2. When you eat out, order a couple of appetizers and skip the main course.

3. With every meal try to have foods that are different in several ways. Have something crunchy, something smooth, something cool and refreshing, something spicy.

4. One easy way to increase variety is to add a low-calorie soup to your menu.

5. Sweets are also part of the variety we crave. Try incorporating a small serving of fruits or low-calorie sweet into most of your meals. This may also reduce your risk of bingeing on sweets (for those of you who have this tendency).

6. Identify your cravings and incorporate that food (or a key aspect of that food) into your next meal or snack. If you find yourself craving a slice of cake, try to figure out what it is that appeals to you about that right then. Is it a desire for something sweet? Then have some fruit or a piece of gum. Is it something smooth that you want? Have low-fat yoghurt or a low-fat ice cream. Something buttery? Try a piece of toast with a scraping of butter. By isolating the quality of the food you crave, you can try to satisfy it with a food that is lower in calories.

7. Remember, what you crave is variety, and your mouth can't tell how much of a food you are eating. Eat a small amount and see if that satisfies you. It often will.

For carbohydrate counters: This type of diet is a real challenge for variety seekers, because at least part of its power comes from the limitation on variety. Even though your selection of foods is very restricted, especially in the early part of the diet, focus on providing yourself with a variety of textures and other sensory aspects of the food.

For calorie counters: This type of diet is really perfect for variety seekers because you can choose any type of food you want. The key for you is going to be portion control. If you don't get the variety you crave, you may still not feel satisfied. You might blame the small portions, but the real problem is insufficient variety.

For fat counters: Carbohydrates are naturally the most diverse of all food groups, so satisfying your need for variety should be relatively easy. Remember to serve yourself small portions, and if you are not satisfied at the end of the meal, consider trying a small portion of another low-calorie food rather than going back for seconds of foods you have already eaten.

RICHNESS

'I come from a family where gravy is considered a beverage.'
— ERMA BOMBECK, COMEDIENNE

If you selected primarily *c*'s under What Makes You Feel Full on the questionnaire, then you respond to the composition of your meals rather than to their size or variety. In general, people like you need to eat meat or some other source of protein to really feel full. You could eat a small steak and feel more full than if you ate a huge salad.

How this works still is not clear, but let me tell you what is known at this point. As background, you need to know that most meals are made up of a combination of carbohydrates, proteins and fats. These comprise what is known as the macronutrient content of food (as opposed to the micronutrient content: vitamins and minerals). Research suggests that each of these three macronutrients has a different ability to reduce hunger.

Protein has been shown to have the greatest ability to reduce hunger. Carbohydrates are next. And fats do very poorly in reducing hunger; they help mainly by making the sensation of fullness last longer. How does this work? As soon as you put food in your mouth, your body is hard at work trying to break the food down into basic components that can then be absorbed into your bloodstream. There are enzymes in your mouth, which start breaking down simple carbohydrates. This is why you can get a sugary taste when you chew something salty for a long time; the amylase in your saliva breaks the cracker carbohydrate down to its most basic component, glucose, while it's still in your mouth. In your stomach and small intestines, enzymes go to work breaking down proteins and fats, and as these are absorbed, your body releases other chemicals to help process the foods.

There is a multitude of these organic chemicals released, but the two most important are cholecystokinin (known as CCK) and insulin. CCK is specifically released in response to the consumption of proteins and fats, and insulin is specifically released in response to proteins and carbohydrates. These two chemicals work with the body to let you know when you have had enough to eat.

They work in a variety of ways. For example, CCK promotes a feeling of fullness by slowing down the rate at which the stomach moves food into the small intestine. Decreasing that rate keeps food in the stomach longer and allows a larger quantity of food to accumulate in the stomach. More food in the stomach is a signal that you have eaten enough. In addition, both CCK and insulin talk directly to the brain to let it know that the right amount of food has been eaten and that it's time to stop eating.

People who respond most strongly to this signal tend to do well on diets that emphasize proteins – either a calorie-counting diet or a carbohydrate-counting diet – because it is easier for them to eat less food overall if they eat more of the foods that make them feel full fastest.

Tips for Those Who Need Richness, No Matter What Diet They Are On

1. Proteins and fats are very sating foods, so serving sizes can be modest.

2. Carbohydrates should always be eaten with a protein in order to help you feel full. I have listed several snacks on page 294 that combine carbs with a protein for a low-fat snack. Each of these snacks has 200 or fewer calories.

3. Those of you who need fat and protein to feel full may want to add nuts to the list of foods you can eat. They are rich in fats and protein, and they are good for you too. But it's easy to overeat nuts. Below are listed the amounts of nuts that make up a snack. I suggest you prepackage them in one-serving helpings. That way, if you overeat, at least you are aware of it.

For calorie counters: Vegetarian cookery books are excellent sources of high-protein meals for calorie counters. *The Good Housekeeping Step by Step Vegetarian Cookbook* (Ebury Press), has a wealth of

ONE-SERVING SNACKS

Nuts or Seeds	Fat (g)	Calories (Kcals)	Carbohydrate (g)
Almonds, 30g (1oz)	17	184	3
Brazils, 40g (1¼oz)	20	205	1
Cashews, 30g (1oz)	14	172	5
Peanuts, 30g (1oz)	14	170	4
Pine nuts, 30g (1oz)	21	206	1
Pistachios, 30g (1oz)	16	180	2

CARB/PROTEIN SNACK COMBINATIONS

Snack	Fat (g)	Calories
Apple and low-fat string cheese	5.5	145
Carrots, celery and 4 tbsp hummus	6	140
Celery stuffed with 1 tbsp cream cheese	10	140
Cucumbers, sliced, and 90g (3oz) low-fat cottage cheese	2	100
Figs (2) and 30g (1oz) prosciutto	5	165
Fruit Smoothie, small (½ recipe from page 221)	1	140
Potato, baked, small, with 2 tbsp low-fat soured cream and salsa	4	205
Strawberries with 240ml (8fl oz) low-fat natural yoghurt	4	190
Tortilla chips, baked, 20 chips, and Pico de Gallo (page 224)	3.5	245

recipes that provide good alternatives to meat as the meal's centre-piece. Also consider cookery books from cultures with a heavily vegetarian population. For example, Indian cuisine features many foods that are high in protein and low in fat, and still provide the richness you seek.

For fat counters: Remember that meat is not the only source of protein in a diet; eggs, dairy products and many vegetables also contain large amounts of protein and should be a major component of the fat counter's diet, since they need protein to feel full. Plan to make one or two meals a week vegetarian so that you can maintain a moderate fat intake on a weekly basis.

DIETING BEHAVIOUR

If you had a score greater than 30 in the How Dieting Changes the Way You Eat section, then you may have dieting behaviours that contribute to your inability to control your weight.

Psychiatrists have identified three attributes of eating behaviour that affect dieters' ability to lose weight and keep it off. The three qualities are:

1. Dietary restraint – the extent to which you try to select foods that are consistent with your dietary goal and reject foods that are not. This is, for example, choosing fruit for dessert rather than a slice of chocolate cake. You allow yourself a dessert, but one that you know has fewer calories.

2. Hunger – your perception of your need for food.

3. Disinhibition – the extent to which you eat, or possibly overeat, in response to the presence of yummy food or other stimuli, such as emotional distress. For example, Janet craves cookies when she gets angry or annoyed at work. When she really wants to yell at someone, she often finds herself at the snack machine wolfing down sweets.

Having restraint makes it easier to lose weight or maintain that new weight. Disinhibition makes both harder – this may seem pretty obvious. But it's actually a little more complicated than that. Many dieters who have high restraint can also have high levels of disinhibition. In fact, this seems to be a particularly common combination in yo-yo dieters. Here is how it works: a high level of restraint is often associated with very rigid attitudes about eating. When something prevents the dieter from eating exactly as she plans, her dietary restraint breaks down, and her disinhibition leads her to eat in a way that is completely *counter* to her ideals. This can sometimes even lead to episodes of bingeing. In other words, if you end up at McDonald's – because you're travelling and arrived after other places closed or because you were late and didn't have a chance to eat but now you just want to grab something quick – you're upset because you're breaking your diet. Because you're upset, you're tempted to overeat once you are there.

What can you do if you have a high level of disinhibition? Awareness is important but not sufficient. In general, the best strategy is to figure out what your triggers are and either avoid them or come up with an alternate plan to the usual eating response. For those dieters who have high levels of restraint and high levels of disinhibition, the goal should be to develop some flexibility in how you think about your diet. When you eat something that is not on your diet, which is inevitable, you need to be careful of how you handle that. The temptation is to say, 'Well, now that I have erred, what the hell. I'll start the diet again tomorrow', and then eat in a disinhibited way. A better alternative is to think, 'Well, I screwed up. Let's try to get back on track, starting now'.

It's easier said than done, as you know. But recognizing these behaviours and working to change them is essential to successful weight-loss maintenance.

BINGE EATING DISORDER

'The belly rules the mind.'
— LATIN PROVERB

If you scored 11 or higher on this section, you may have binge eating disorder. Doctors increasingly recognize that a small but significant minority of overweight individuals struggle with episodes of massive overeating. Overeaters Anonymous popularized the most widely used term for this – compulsive overeating. Psychiatrists call this binge eating disorder.

This disorder is characterized by episodes of uncontrolled eating during which the individual feels that she has lost control of her ability to stop. She may eat large quantities of food and not stop until she feels uncomfortably, painfully full. These individuals binge frequently – as much as twice a week and often more. These binges occur when alone, and an episode of bingeing is usually followed by feelings of guilt and self-loathing. Obviously, individuals with this disorder have more difficulty losing weight and keeping it off. Most of them are obese and have a history of weight fluctuations.

There is a variation of binge eating that has been recently recognized, called night eating syndrome. In this disorder, individuals consume more than 50 per cent of their total caloric intake at night, often eating when they are unable to fall asleep or even waking up at night and bingeing before going back to bed.

If you think that you may have one of these disorders, do yourself a big favour and talk to your doctor about it. The presence of these problems makes losing weight particularly difficult. Many people with binge eating disorder can be helped through talk therapy or structured weight-loss programmes that address their particular needs. Overeaters Anonymous is also recommended by many experts in the field, although there is no published data on this group's success rate. You need to recognize this problem and find the assistance you need in order to manage your weight.

CHAPTER 11

MEDICAL HISTORY

THE MOST IMPORTANT REASON for changing your diet and losing weight is to help you become healthier. Of course, even though the majority of us are trying to lose weight, the goal, far too often, is simply to look good. Luckily, so long as you choose a reasonable diet, the health benefits are automatic.

In fact, you don't even have to lose weight to see many of the benefits from what we think of as dieting. Simply choosing your food carefully and increasing your activity level – those things that most of us mean when we say we are on a diet – can dramatically improve your health and lengthen your life. When you actually lose weight and bring yourself closer to a BMI of less than 26, the health benefits really start to roll in. A 10 per cent weight loss will go a long way towards fixing what ails you. It will bring down your blood pressure (if it's too high), reduce your cholesterol, improve your blood sugar and insulin, and reduce your risk of developing diabetes or heart disease.

Your target weight is a personal decision based on how you want to look and feel, and I can't tell you what you should weigh. This much I *can* tell you, though: a loss of 5 to 10 per cent of your weight will help you feel better, be healthier and live longer. When people say that diets don't work, they are talking about how hard it is for many, and maybe for most, of us to reach what we feel is our ideal weight. But, even if you never achieve that elusive goal, the one way that diets can work is by making you healthier.

On the other hand, many of us have at least one health problem that can be improved by how we eat, and that is what this chapter is all about. I've tried to condense this important information to make it as accessible as possible, to give you concrete suggestions on modifying your diet to address your health needs as you lose weight. But of course, before you start on this (or any) diet programme, you should consult your doctor. Successful weight loss will have an effect on many health problems, and you may need to adjust your medications as you progress towards your goal.

YOUR MEDICAL HISTORY

If you have a score of 3 or greater in this section of the questionnaire, then you may be at increased risk of developing heart disease. In general, cardiac risk factors are divided into those which are modifiable (those which have to do with lifestyle and the development and treatment of chronic disease) and those which are not (primarily sex and age).

In general, older individuals are at higher risk than younger, and men are at risk at a younger age than women. You can't do much about these factors, so let's move on to those you can influence. In this section, I will tell you what the research shows that you should be eating – or not as the case may be – if you have any of these underlying medical conditions.

Smoking

Not exactly news to anyone, but smoking is bad for you. What may surprise you, however, is that most smokers don't die of lung cancer, nor do most smokers die of emphysema. The vast majority of smokers die from heart disease.

A common reason for not quitting smoking is fear of weight gain. The average amount of weight gained during smoking cessation is 2.75kg (6lb). On the other hand, once you quit smoking it's easier to lose weight, because it's easier to live an active life, and that helps with weight loss.

It is hard to quit. (I quit after smoking for 15 years, and I still consider that to be one of the great achievements of my life.) But it can be done. Research suggests that the use of a nicotine-replacement device – either the patch, the inhaler or the gum – plus the use of Zyban prior to quitting is a pretty successful combo.

Those of you who aren't yet able to quit (I wouldn't be much of a doctor if I didn't think there was always hope) should address the other cardiac risk factors that place you at higher risk. Below I've listed some of the ways diet can help you with this.

In addition, smokers as well as former smokers may be able to reduce their risk of developing lung cancer by eating a diet high in fruits and vegetables. In some studies, smokers who ate a diet rich in fruits and vegetables (more than five servings per day) decreased their risk of lung cancer by a third.

You might be tempted to skip the fruits and vegetables and just take beta-carotene, vitamin E or other antioxidants in pill form. Don't do it. When studies compared smokers who took these supplements with those who did not, taking the antioxidants actually *increased* the cancer, rather than reducing it. And in participants who ate lots of fruits and veggies and took antioxidants, the two interventions cancelled each other out – so they were at the same risk as those who did neither. In addition, a diet rich in omega fats may also reduce your risk of lung cancer and heart disease. In a study done in Greece, which has one of the highest rates of smoking in the world, men who ate the traditional Mediterranean diet – rich in fruits, vegetables and fish – lived much longer than those who did not.

Bottom line: quitting smoking is the most effective way to improve your health. Even if you can't quit (yet), a diet high in fruits, vegetables and seafood will reduce your risk of dying from smoking-related disease.

Cholesterol

As you probably know by now, there are several different types of cholesterol that should be measured by your doctor. A quick refresher about each of them. First, there is the so-called bad cholesterol, LDL. This is the form of cholesterol most highly correlated with risk of heart attack or stroke. Healthy people should have an LDL cholesterol level of less than 3 millimoles per litre of blood (mmol/L). People who have either diabetes or have had heart disease in the past and so are at a higher risk of heart disease should have an LDL cholesterol level of less than 2.6 mmol/L.

HDL cholesterol is the so-called good cholesterol. Having high HDL is associated with a lower risk of heart disease. Men should have an HDL level of greater than 1.0 mmol/L, and women, who naturally have a somewhat higher level of HDL, should have an HDL level of greater than 1.1 mmol/L. Then there are triglycerides, the storage form of fat – your triglyceride level should be less than 2.0 mmol/L. Finally, there is total cholesterol. That is a measured value that takes LDL, HDL and triglycerides into consideration. Having a total cholesterol level of less than 5.0 mmol/L is associated with a lower risk of heart disease.

So what should you do if your cholesterol is outside the healthy range? The recommendations change based on which type of cholesterol is abnormal.

LDL and total cholesterol. I lump these two together because elevated total cholesterol is usually due to elevated LDL cholesterol. (On occasion, it's due to elevated HDL, and that is a good thing, so you don't need to do anything except keep up the good work.) The best way to bring down your LDL cholesterol is to eat a diet lower in saturated fat.

Exercise plus a diet low in saturated and trans fats is the best way to bring down your LDL cholesterol. Not only does it reduce the amount of LDL in your blood, but the LDL that remains is less likely to cause heart disease.

Bottom line: if your LDL is too high, cut the amount of saturated and trans fats in your diet.

HDL cholesterol. Since this is the good cholesterol, in general, the more HDL you have, the better off you are. Increasing the amount of good fat in your diet will increase HDL. By good fat, I mean, of course, not the fat from meats but that from plants and seeds and seafood. Polyunsaturated fats, corn oil, for example, as well as monounsaturated fats (olive oil or rapeseed oil) will bring up HDL. And omega fatty acids found in seafood will too. Eating saturated fats from meat will increase your HDL but will increase your LDL as well, so they cancel each other out. Exercise will also help increase your good cholesterol. Current research suggests that this occurs primarily by reducing insulin resistance. (For more information on insulin resistance, check out the section on metabolic syndrome on page 309.)

Modest consumption of alcohol will elevate your HDL. It's not a reason to take up drinking, but it is one more reason to enjoy the occasional glass of wine if you already drink.

Oestrogen increases HDL levels; that's why women have a

higher baseline HDL than men, at least before menopause. And it was one of the reasons that hormone therapy after menopause was advocated in the last century, but it didn't work. Researchers found that women on hormone therapy who were taking oestrogen plus progesterone had a slightly higher rate of heart disease than women who didn't. Health food stores are trying to promote eating natural oestrogens found in plants – they're called phytoestrogens – using the argument that these foods or drugs will increase HDL levels. They may, but it's clear that the relationship between oestrogen and heart disease isn't a straightforward 'more-is-less' type of deal. More research is needed on this topic before phytoestrogens can be medically recommended.

Bottom line: a diet rich in good fats and low in bad fats is the best way to increase your HDL. Alcohol and exercise also increase HDL.

Triglycerides. Finally, let's talk about triglycerides. These are maybe the most interesting part of the whole lipid profile and have only got attention very recently. They are the storage form of fats in your body. Plain fat is hydrophobic and doesn't mix well with water. In triglycerides, fats are linked to a carbohydrate backbone, and that allows them to deal with the watery world of our bodies. Fat deposits throughout the body are basically stockpiles of triglycerides. Mostly, those stay put. There are triglycerides in the blood as well. These are fats on their way somewhere – either to be used by the cells or stored in fat deposits.

Here's what's interesting about triglycerides: for many people, the amount of triglycerides in the blood is due not to how much fat was in the most recent meal, but how much carbohydrate. That's right: triglyceride levels increase after a meal high in carbohydrates. Pretty amazing. Although the exact physiology of this phenomenon hasn't been completely worked out, it looks as though the people most likely to have this tendency are those with insulin resistance.

Given the link between triglycerides, insulin resistance and heart disease, it is important that those with high triglycerides eat a diet relatively high in good fats and stick to whole grain carbohydrates and other foods with a low glycaemic load. What this means is that you should replace potatoes and starches in your diet with nuts, olive oil and seafood, which contain good fats, and fruits, vegetables and whole grains (brown bread rather than white bread; old-fashioned porridge over instant; beans rather than pasta) to maximally reduce your triglycerides.

Diabetes

This disease increases the risk of heart disease dramatically, because having elevated glucose levels damages the blood vessels and makes it easier for people with diabetes to develop narrowed arteries in the heart and throughout the body. Because of this increased risk of heart disease, other risk factors like high blood pressure, high cholesterol and smoking have to be well-managed.

How people with diabetes should eat has been the source of much controversy over the past few decades. Initially, it was thought that they should avoid sweets and sugar. As understanding of carbohydrate metabolism grew, and it was understood that all carbohydrates turn to sugar in the body, all carbohydrates were declared equal, and the move was towards spreading them throughout the day to achieve predictable and controllable blood sugar levels, even in the hour or so after eating a meal.

Until recently, people with diabetes were almost universally put on low-fat, high-carbohydrate diets because of concerns about the elevated cardiac risk they faced. Now there is some movement away from the low-fat diet to one that allows more fat and fewer carbohydrates.

The carbohydrates that are eaten should have a low glycaemic load. This means choosing fruits and vegetables over starches and breads. People with diabetes should not necessarily decrease the total amount of fat in their diets but should chose more mono- and poly-unsaturated fats and omega fats instead of saturated fat. In practice, this means more lean meat and fish, more nuts and olive oil. And fewer starches – less pasta, less rice and fewer potatoes, but more vegetables. If this sounds a lot like the advice given to those with low HDL and those with high triglycerides, it is. And that's because all three problems – diabetes, low HDL and high triglycerides – are caused by the same underlying factor: insulin resistance. So you shouldn't be surprised that the treatment is the same. They are all aspects of the same underlying defect.

Weight loss will improve insulin resistance. A brisk 30-minute walk 5 days a week will help keep your sugars in line. Losing 10 per cent of your weight will improve your blood pressure, lower your cholesterol and improve your glycaemic control.

Daily goals for blood glucose should be readings between 4 and 7 mmol/l before meals and readings of less than 10 mmol/l after meals. Long-term control of glucose is adequate when the result of your HbA1c blood test – that's the measure of long-term glucose control – is less than 6.5 per cent.

High Blood Pressure

For most people, normal blood pressure is less than 140/90 millimetres of mercury (mm Hg). People with diabetes or serious kidney disease should aim for a blood pressure even lower than that: 125/80. Elevated blood pressure can increase risk of stroke, heart disease and kidney disease.

Doctors could measure blood pressure and had known its risks long before we had any medicines for treating it. At that point, diet and lifestyle change were really the only tools we had to combat this deadly disease. (Sound familiar?) The tendency to develop high blood pressure is inherited. If one or both of your parents had high blood pressure, you are at pretty high risk of developing it as well. Even so, biology is not destiny. So what lowers blood pressure? Just about everything that's good for you: exercising daily, reducing your weight, eating more fruits and vegetables, and finally, reducing your sodium intake (the vast majority of the sodium we ingest comes from salt so this basically means eating less salt).

How do you moderate your salt intake? Good question. I frequently challenge my students to try to lower their salt intake just so they'll appreciate firsthand how tough this is. Salt is everywhere. The salt you put *on* your food is just a drop in the bucket of what makes its way into your body every day.

Salt is an important preservative and a convenient way for manufacturers to add flavour to processed foods. So virtually everything that is processed is loaded with salt. If they take the salt out, the food doesn't taste like anything at all.

So, here's how to follow a low-salt diet: avoid prepared foods. This includes prepared meals that are chilled, frozen or that come in cans. These foods can contain a surprisingly large amount of salt – a ready-made supermarket lasagne, for example, can contain up to 4.5 grams of salt. Most packaged foods will list the amount of sodium – to convert this figure to salt, multiply it by 2.5.

What's the right amount of salt in a low-salt diet? A low-salt diet is generally defined as one in which no more than 4 grams (the equivalent of 1.6 grams of sodium) of table salt are consumed per day. The current average intake is thought to be between 9 and 12 grams so the necessary reduction is a significant one. The only way to achieve this is to eat primarily fresh foods and have the only salt in your food be what you add for flavour.

It's a challenge. And a very tough goal when so many of us depend on prepackaged foods at home and eat out frequently. Nevertheless, studies have shown that sticking to a low-sodium diet brings blood pressure down significantly. For many people, it can make the difference between having to take high blood pressure medication or not. Try it. Keep track of where your salt comes from and see if you can bring it down.

So here's how to follow a low-sodium diet.

1. Avoid prepared foods.
2. Avoid foods that are canned, cured (like bacon), pickled (in brine) or smoked (ham).
3. Avoid condiments such as MSG (monosodium glutamate), ketchup and mustard.
4. Don't add salt to the cooking water for vegetables, rice or pasta.
5. Rinse canned foods to remove some of the sodium.
6. Buy low-sodium canned or prepackaged foods.

Bottom line: if you have high blood pressure, eat a diet rich in fruits and vegetables and low in sodium, and exercise as often as you can.

Heart Disease

Once you have had a heart attack or angina or an angioplasty, your cardiologist will very likely encourage you to see a nutritionist to help you change the way you eat. The nutritionist will probably want you to go on a low-fat, high-carbohydrate diet. A fat-counting diet, which dramatically limits saturated fats, has been shown to reverse heart disease.

Is that the best diet for those with heart disease? Not necessarily. Any diet that restricts saturated fat and cholesterol and emphasizes fresh vegetables, whole grains and fish will lower your risk of having a second heart attack. The Mediterranean diet, as it has come to be known, fits this bill. Based on the Seven Countries study done in seven Mediterranean countries associated with a lower risk of heart disease, this diet emphasizes fresh fruits and vegetables, olive oil and other monounsaturated fats, fish and chicken over beef, whole grains over processed flours, and moderate consumption of wine.

A 4-year study compared this diet to the low-fat diet normally recommended and found that the Mediterranean diet was associated with a 50 per cent reduction in risk of a second heart attack. So, even after a heart attack, there is choice about how to change your diet to improve your health, while still finding one you can enjoy and stick to. Here are some tips on how to eat if you have heart disease.

1. Incorporate nuts into your daily eating plan. These are a great source of protein and good fats.

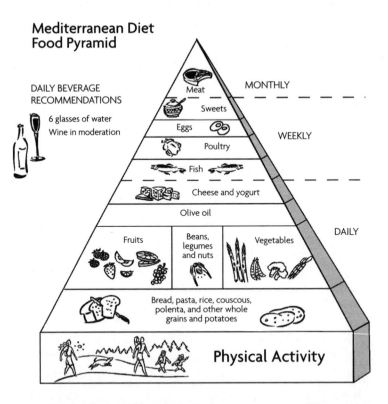

Mediterranean Diet Food Pyramid

DAILY BEVERAGE RECOMMENDATIONS

6 glasses of water
Wine in moderation

Meat — MONTHLY

Sweets

Eggs

Poultry — WEEKLY

Fish

Cheese and yogurt

Olive oil

Fruits | Beans, legumes and nuts | Vegetables — DAILY

Bread, pasta, rice, couscous, polenta, and other whole grains and potatoes

Physical Activity

© 2000 Oldways Preservation & Exchange Trust   www.oldwayspt.org

2. Make sure the carbohydrates you eat are low-glycaemic-load foods. Aim for foods with a glycaemic load of less than 20. This means more fruits and vegetables, wholemeal breads and crackers, with few pastries, biscuits and breads made from refined flour.

3. Many low-fat meals centre on a starchy carbohydrate; these foods tend to have a higher glycaemic load than fruits and vegetables. Because of this, you should reduce the amount of starchy carbohydrates (like rice, noodles or pasta) and increase the amount of fruits and vegetables. Cutting the starch in half and doubling the other ingredients will help you control your insulin levels.

4. Make most of the meat that you eat fish and other seafood.

5. When you do eat meat, make sure you choose the leanest meats with more poultry than pork, more pork than beef.

6. When you eat dairy products, make sure you are eating the low-fat version.

7. Avoid trans fats. Check food labels for the presence of partially hydrogenated oils, and if it has them, don't buy it.

8. Watch your calories.

METABOLIC SYNDROME

If you scored 3 points or higher on the section about metabolic syndrome, then you have it – but you shouldn't feel alone. Researchers estimate it affects 5 million people in the UK.

So what is metabolic syndrome? It is a group of abnormalities that tend to run together and dramatically increase an individual's risk of heart disease. This phenomenon was first described in 1988 by Gerald Reaven, MD, an endocrinologist at Stanford University who noticed that many of his patients who had high blood pressure also had diabetes, or at least a higher-than-normal blood glucose level. Also, many of them had trunkal obesity – that is, they carried their excess weight predominately around their waists. Plus, many of them also had abnormal cholesterol with elevated triglyceride levels and low levels of HDL.

All of these problems were linked by a single cause: their bodies were resistant to the effects of what is probably the most complex and important hormone in our bodies: insulin. Most people have heard about insulin because some people with diabetes don't have enough of it and must inject it in order to live. That's because one of insulin's most important jobs (though not by any means its only job) is to help cells take up glucose from the bloodstream. People who have insulin resistance need much higher levels of insulin to get that job done, but high levels of insulin can be problematic.

For example, high levels of insulin cause the body to hold on to salt, which in turn makes the body hold on to water, which can cause high blood pressure. High insulin also encourages fat to accumulate around your waist. Abdominal fat is the most metabolically active fat; that means that it is the easiest to put on and the easiest to take off. So if you lose weight, you will probably lose at least some of that fat. That's the good news. The bad news is that abdominal fat is associated with higher rates of cardiac disease.

High insulin levels also help turn carbohydrates into fats.

All this adds up to a higher risk of heart disease. How much higher? It looks as if it could increase your odds of having heart disease by as much as 400 per cent. If you are under 35 and a woman, your risk of having a heart attack is very low, so an increase of 400 per cent, while it sounds scary, probably doesn't increase your real risk of a heart attack very much. But if you are a woman approaching menopause or a man, then your baseline risk is greater, and a 400 per cent increase can really make a difference.

The tendency to develop insulin resistance is inherited. It's not like having blue eyes, where you either have it or you don't. It's the *tendency* to develop insulin resistance, like the tendency to be a good athlete. The possibility is there, but you have to do certain things for it to develop. It's nature plus nurture. So what can nurture this trait? Obesity can. Not everyone with insulin resistance is overweight, but if you are overweight and have this inborn predisposition, it will bring it out.

Having a sedentary lifestyle will too. Muscles play an important role in taking glucose up out of the blood. If they are not being used, they don't take up as much glucose, and somehow that sets the stage for insulin resistance.

If there are factors that promote the development of insulin resistance and metabolic syndrome, are there factors that reduce the likelihood of developing it? There are. Exercise is the most powerful factor, and it's surprising how little you need for therapeutic effect. A brisk daily walk lasting half an hour will reduce the likelihood by almost 50 per cent. What you eat also makes a difference in whether or not you develop insulin resistance. A diet rich in whole grains and fruits and vegetables and low in sugary drinks is associated with a lower risk. A high-fibre diet is also associated with a lower risk of developing metabolic syndrome. And finally, and perhaps most surprisingly, a diet rich in dairy products is associated with a much lower risk of developing metabolic syndrome.

Of course, if you are reading this, chances are you already have metabolic syndrome. So now what? In general, the same things that reduce your chance of developing metabolic syndrome will also help you get rid of it by reducing your level of insulin resistance. So, weight loss will certainly reverse much of the insulin resistance you have developed. One more reason to keep trying to achieve the proper weight. But until then, eating a diet that is high in fibre, high in low-fat dairy products, and high in whole grains and vegetables will help. Exercise also is extremely helpful in fighting insulin resistance.

One last thing: if you have metabolic syndrome with high triglycerides, then you should probably avoid the low-fat, high-carbohydrate diet. Individuals with insulin resistance have this amazing ability to turn carbohydrates into fats. Dr Reaven, the endocrinologist who first described metabolic syndrome, recommends a diet high in monounsaturated fats (like those in olive oil, rapeseed oil and nuts) and relatively low in carbohydrates.

Dr Reaven's perfect diet would include 40 per cent of daily calories from monounsaturated fats and about the same from carbohydrates. Moreover, the carbs that you do eat should be fruits and vegetables or whole grains. Refined carbohydrates should be avoided. They turn rapidly into glucose once you eat them and promote the release of high levels of insulin, and that only makes the whole business worse.

Bottom line: if you have metabolic syndrome, you should follow these guidelines.

1. Eat a diet high in monounsaturated fats. (For more information on what kinds of foods are high in monounsaturated fats, see 'Know Your Fats' page 242.)
2. Eat fruits and vegetables daily.
3. Avoid refined carbohydrates.
4. Eat a diet rich in low-fat or reduced-fat dairy products.
5. Try to get 30 minutes of exercise every day.

FAMILY MEDICAL HISTORY

If your parents had heart disease at an early age, or any of the associated risk factors of heart disease – diabetes, high blood pressure or high cholesterol – then you are at risk of developing these diseases as well.

A heart attack before the age of 45 in a man or 55 in a woman is an unusual event – though not nearly unusual enough. If your mother or father had one, then that increases the chance that you will develop heart disease as well. How much that risk is increased isn't known, but a family history of heart disease at an early age is a signal that risk factors should be screened for and well-controlled to reduce that risk as much as possible.

If one of your parents had diabetes, then you are also at risk of developing diabetes. Fortunately, being at risk doesn't mean you will – it means you could. A study published in *The New England Journal of Medicine* in 2002 showed that even people at very high risk of developing diabetes – those with insulin resistance – could prevent that by losing some weight and exercising. The participants in this study lost 7 per cent of their initial body weight over the course of 6 months and kept most of that off. Losing that much weight prevented most of them from developing diabetes. People in the study were asked to engage in moderate exercise (they sweat lightly but were still able to talk) for 150 minutes a week, just over 20 minutes a day.

If you have a family history of diabetes, you can dramatically reduce your risk of developing diabetes as well by maintaining a healthy weight and exercising daily. When I talk about diabetes, I am talking about what is called adult onset diabetes, or type 2 diabetes, which can be treated with pills as well as insulin. The other type of diabetes – juvenile, or type 1, diabetes – must always be treated with insulin, and does not run in families.

What about high blood pressure? All of us are at risk of developing high blood pressure eventually. Half of everyone over the age of 60 has it. If either of your parents have high blood pressure then you too are at a higher risk of developing it as well. What can you do to reduce or prevent it? The answers are probably what you would expect.

1. Lose weight. In one study an average weight loss of just 3.6kg (8lb) cut the risk of developing high blood pressure in half.

2. Reduce salt intake. Researchers found that cutting salt to less than 6 grams per day dropped blood pressure by an average of 3 mm Hg. That may not sound like much to you, but in one long-term population study, a 2 mm Hg drop in blood pressure reduced the risk of developing high blood pressure by 20 per cent.

3. Exercise. Moderate exercise done 30 minutes per day, most days of the week, will reduce blood pressure by 4 mm Hg.

4. Reduce your alcohol intake. A number of studies have shown that reducing alcohol intake to no more than two drinks per day for men and one drink per day for women lowered blood pressure by 4 mm Hg.

5. Eat a diet high in potassium. Eating bananas, oranges or leafy greens daily was associated with a 2 mm Hg drop in blood pressure.

6. Eat a diet rich in fruits, fresh vegetables and low-fat dairy products and low in saturated fats. This diet was associated with a 4 mm Hg drop in blood pressure.

Finally, what about cholesterol? If you have a family history of high cholesterol, then you may be at risk of high cholesterol yourself. Obviously, diet is a major contributor in the development of high cholesterol, but your genes speak here as well. It is advisable for all adults aged 20 or over to have their cholesterol measured.

This is a much younger age at which to start screening than was previously recommended, so if you are under the age of 40, you may not have had your cholesterol checked. You should discuss this with your doctor and see if she wants to measure it now.

Certainly if you have a family history of high cholesterol or early heart disease or if you have diabetes, you should seriously consider having your cholesterol checked at regular intervals.

Your risk of developing high cholesterol if you have a family history of it isn't clear at this point. But even if you don't have high cholesterol now, you should certainly consider eating a diet low in saturated fat and cholesterol in that setting. Diet alone can bring down cholesterol 10 to 15 per cent on average, and that may be all you really need at this point. For more information on how to eat a low-saturated-fat diet, see chapter 9.

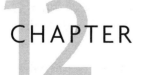

CHAPTER

FAMILY HERITAGE

YOUR FAMILY INHERITANCE: NATURE

If you scored 5 or more in the section titled How You Are Shaped by Nature, there is a good chance that you have inherited traits from your family that make controlling your weight difficult. It's easy to imagine that a tendency to gain weight is as inherited as having red hair or being tall or having broad shoulders. Recent studies have put a finer point on it: genes govern not only where you put on weight but also how you get fat. That is to say, it's not just the body that gets handed down to you, but the behaviour you're likely use to run it as well.

Most of us observe something among our friends when we're young. If the parents of a family are overweight, then the kids are more likely to be overweight too. It used to be thought that this was due to the shared environment: you were taught about food and how to eat by your parents. If they overate, they would teach you to overeat as well. The environment does play a powerful role, but research done within the past two decades suggests that there is also a strong genetic component.

Dr Albert Stunkard, one of the pioneers in the science of obesity, asked this question: Is the tendency to gain weight inherited or learned? He then looked at children who were adopted and compared their weights to the weights of both their adopted and biological parents. He found that the adopted children were much more likely to have the same body-weight class as their biological parents rather than their adopted parents. It wasn't true in 100 per cent of cases, but it was significant. Much more than would be expected if it were just a coincidence.

Then Dr Stunkard asked another question: How big a role did genes play? In order to answer this question, he looked at obesity in identical and fraternal twins. Identical twins share the exact same genes. Fraternal twins share exactly half the same set of genes. (The same as any two siblings would.) Dr Stunkard looked at twins who were raised together and compared them with twins raised separately. If some certain trait showed up more commonly among identical twins than in fraternal twins, then it would seem obvious that the trait was more likely due to their genes rather than their environment. That's the theory, and twin studies have been used extensively in figuring out what is nature, or inborn, and what is nurture, or learned.

In Europe it's easy to find twins. You simply contact – I'm not making this up – the Swedish Twins Registry. There are about 25,000 twins on file there, so Dr Stunkard tracked down about 600 pairs of twins born between 1886 and 1958. Of these, about 100 were identical twins who were raised in the same home and 100 were identical twins raised apart. He also located 200 fraternal pairs raised together and 200 who were raised separately. Then he compared the body mass indexes (BMIs) of each twin pair.

He found that the twins who were raised together were more likely to have the same bodies. So environment does count. But he also found that fraternal twins raised apart were likely to share the same body shape. And here's what's most surprising: more than two-thirds of the identical twins who were raised apart had the same BMI.

So there is clearly a very important genetic component to weight gain. But how does a genetic predisposition express itself?

One genetic trait is how well you burn off calories. Although there aren't big differences in basic metabolic rates, there is a difference in how active people are. And I'm not referring to whether you are an athlete or not, but to the activity of daily life. Whether you are a toe-tapping fidgeter or a serene Buddha is an inherited quality. And fidgeters burn off more calories than those who are able to sit still. Still, it's not a lot of calories and certainly can't account for all of the weight.

So researchers started looking at eating behaviours and asked the question, are these behaviours inherited? Food preference was known to have some inherited quality – sensitivity to bitter foods has been well-described (see page 277 for information about those who have this sensitivity), but its link to obesity was not clear. So once again researchers turned to twins to answer that question.

American researchers recruited 2,300 pairs of twins over the age of 50 (they had to advertise for them). Each of the twins filled out a questionnaire about what he or she ate. The researchers then divided the eaters into one of two broad categories: those who ate lots of veggies and whole grains (your basic healthy diet) and those who ate lots of fats and sweets (your basic all-American, unhealthy diet). And then they compared the twins to see how often they fell into the same pattern-of-eating category.

There was no pattern in the unhealthy dieters. Whether they were identical twins or fraternal twins didn't matter. And, curiously, none of the women seemed to show the effect of any genetic influence. But men who ate a healthy diet did show evidence of a genetic component: if one of the identical twin men had a healthy pattern of eating, there was a very good chance that his brother did too. Fraternal twins had about half as much a chance as the identical twins. So there does appear to be a genetic component in food choice, especially the (now) unusual choice to eat a healthy diet.

What all this means is that, while there is a genetic component to food preference, it may not be powerful enough to overcome the cultural pressures to eat in a less healthy way. There are other eating behaviours that seem to have a genetic component to them, like disinhibition, or the inability to put on the eating brakes when set off by some trigger – a food you really like or even seeing someone else overeat, for example. You'd think this behaviour was learned, but not according to a study done on a large Amish population in Pennsylvania, chosen because it was socially isolated and the family tree was well-known back to the 18th century. Researchers interviewed hundreds of Amish people from 65 families whose kinship was well-known, and tracing these families back, scientists found that disinhibition was much more likely to run in families than not.

Is biology destiny? Or as one of my patients put it, 'Am I destined to be fat like my parents and sisters?' Obviously, the answer is no. Not every identical twin ended up the same; genetics is only one component of who we are and how we live.

On the other hand, life is not fair. I'm telling you about the role of genetics so that you'll understand that when it comes to gaining weight or losing it, we are not all playing on the same level field. Genes definitely make it harder for some people to gain weight or to lose it. That doesn't mean you should be defeatist or fatalistic about losing weight if the genetic deck seems stacked against you. It means you have to understand where you have an advantage or disadvantage, and take that into account when you're designing your weight-management programme.

It's just harder for some people to lose weight than it is for others. You know it. I know it. And now doctors know it too. That's why your diet and your lifestyle have to be tailored to fit you. One size doesn't fit all, because it doesn't take into consideration all the ways in which we are different. If you can figure out what works for you and you alone, the hardest part of your work will be done.

YOUR FAMILY INHERITANCE: NURTURE

If you scored 15 points or more in the section called How You Are Shaped by Nurture, then your experiences with food and activity as a child may be contributing to your difficulties in managing your weight as an adult.

In this section, we look at your family's attitude towards food and exercise, because there is evidence that these attitudes, shaped early in life, can influence how you feel about food and exercise as an adult.

Let's talk about food first. The way food was made available in your childhood can have an impact on the way you view food as an adult.

Kids up to the age of 3 are able to regulate how much food they eat based on internal cues of satiety. After that point, though, external cues become more important: external cues such as serving size and parental expectations.

Attitudes about food are developed early in life. Many of my patients report having food used as a reward for achievement or a treatment for psychic or physical ills, and for many of them these links have persisted into adulthood. After a long day at work, Janet feels that she 'deserves' a big bowl of ice cream as a reward. And when she doesn't have it, she feels punished, deprived. It has been a struggle for her to address this sense that food is a reward. I hear this over and over again from my patients and my friends: food is a reward, a comfort, therapy.

This sense of food is learned, of course, but on a biological level, food is literally a reward. Voltaire recognized this as early as the 18th century when he said, 'Nothing would be more tiresome than eating and drinking if God had not made them a pleasure as well as a necessity.' Eating and drinking are two of the most primal pleasures that we have – right up there with sex and sleeping.

But food, the easiest legitimate trigger in our culture to obtain and indulge, is not the only thing that tickles our pleasure centres. Many other activities do as well. Exercise is the most widely touted and probably the best. The various magazines devoted to these pursuits still print articles that describe all the hormonal changes that take place in the body when it exercises, the great feelings that surge after a workout, and the near-spiritual quality of the 'endorphin high'. Hobbies and other pursuits can also trigger our pleasure centres. Studies done on recreational activities, even though as ordinary as sewing or gardening, show that they can lower heart rates and blood pressure and tickle our endorphins. Meditation has many of the same effects as opiates except that it doesn't interfere with our ability to drive, make us drool, or make us say things to our friends that provoke head-slapping remorse the next morning.

Our link between food and pleasure is obvious; it's reinforced biologically at least three times a day and often explicitly used as a reward from early childhood. The other pleasure triggers aren't as well-established for us. Few of us were taught to meditate as children to help us cope with the stresses of life. Not when there were biscuits at hand. So, many of us are forced to try to reprogramme this link ourselves as adults. It can be done. It's just a little harder.

One of the ways we make the link between other activities and pleasure is by engaging in them as a family. Families who pursue pleasurable activities together, like sports or hiking or gardening or fishing, are teaching kids about other ways to get rewards. The only thing my family did together was to eat, and our Sunday dinners were without a doubt the best part of our week. But there were two activities my mother did with me and my sisters: she took us to the public library every Saturday, and she taught us how to sew. And to this day, both reading and sewing remain two of my favourite activities.

Exercise that starts early in life has a greater chance of remaining pleasurable and important to us as adults. Few things in life are better at predicting an active adulthood as participating in sports or other physical activities in childhood. But if you didn't learn a sport or hobby as a child, you aren't doomed; it's never too late. It's part of the baggage you brought from childhood, and it has to be unloaded. You are not just the child your parents wanted you to be. As an adult, you have made decisions about who you wanted to be and what you wanted to do that were based on your own needs, desires and goals. The genetic and environmental baggage that you were saddled with as a kid does not determine who you are now.

Learn to recognize childhood habits that are ingrained in your attitudes about food and exercise. Then resolve to reshape those attitudes into ones that are more compatible with your adult goals – with who you are and what you want to do with your life and your body now.

Nature isn't destiny; nurture isn't destiny. They do have an impact on how hard your row is to hoe – to deny that would be to ignore what science tells us. But neither do they determine what can and can't be done. Only we can determine that.

CHAPTER 13
EATING HABITS

Ｆ YOU HAVE A SCORE OF 10 OR MORE in the Eating Habits section of
the questionnaire, chances are good that how you eat is contributing to your difficulty in losing weight or maintaining your
weight.

Welcome to the club. Science has only recently tried to figure out
how the way that we eat affects our ability to maintain our ideal
weight.

In this section of the questionnaire, I look at several aspects of
your eating habits: skipping meals, snacking between meals and
hunger. As you can see, these are very different (albeit related) topics,
and it's not hard to imagine that they may affect whether you gain or
lose weight, although how they do that may surprise you. Later in
the chapter, we'll look at the roles played by emotions and habit in
eating.

SKIPPING MEALS

When I ask patients how they are trying to lose weight, I find that a common strategy is to skip meals or to eat only one meal per day. You know what? It doesn't work. Many of my patients tell me that they don't eat breakfast. By skipping breakfast they figure they will be able to consume fewer calories during the day, because they will be eating only two meals rather than three. That's the theory.

Here's the reality: in multiple studies done in a variety of populations, people who eat breakfast are much less likely to be overweight than people who don't.

Some of my patients tell me that they are not hungry at breakfast time, and that may well be true. There are aspects of meal scheduling and hunger that are learned; that's why we are hungry every 4 to 5 hours during the day but can go for 8 hours overnight as we sleep. If you are out of the habit of breakfast, you will not get hungry for it. Once you start, however, you will find yourself anticipating the meal and getting hungry for it as you do for your other meals.

The other comment I hear from some people is that they get hungry just a couple of hours after eating breakfast and feel as though they stay hungry for the rest of the morning. This is, I think, more a function of what they eat for breakfast than the fact that they are eating breakfast. Commonly, people who complain of this grab a croissant, muffin or toast and coffee. This breakfast may, in fact, make you hungry just a couple of hours later, because it's not very much to eat, and it doesn't stick around very long. Foods containing only refined flour and maybe some fat contain a lot of calories but aren't very satiating.

However, despite not providing much in the way of satisfaction, they're crammed with calories. A croissant spread with butter and jam, for instance, can contain around 450 calories. According to my patients (as well as my own extensive personal experience), a couple of hours after eating a typical refined carbohydrate breakfast, you find yourself at the snack machine eyeing a bag of crisps, just a little something to tide you over until lunchtime.

So, what should you eat for breakfast? Well, in a survey of 122 healthy older men and women in Madrid, Spain, those who were a normal weight ate a more varied breakfast, eating from both a greater number of foods and more groups of foods. They also spent a longer time eating their breakfasts and consumed greater quantities of food than did their overweight counterparts.

So eating a variety of foods and eating enough food is good. A more specific recommendation depends on your diet and the foods you like. In general, I tend to recommend either a high-fibre cereal with fruit and maybe a piece of toast with peanut butter or, if you are counting carbohydrates, something that provides protein with a minimal amount of saturated fat – maybe a poached egg with a couple of slices of back bacon. Just look at the amount of food and the calories compared to that croissant with butter and jam.

40g (1¼oz) All-Bran with skimmed milk	120 calories
1 slice of toast with 1 teaspoon peanut butter	135 calories
½ cantaloupe melon	100 calories
Total	355 calories

How about eggs?

Omelette or scrambled eggs made with 2 whole eggs and 1 egg white	185 calories
30g (1oz) cheese, added to the omelette	115 calories
2 slices of back bacon	90 calories
Total	390 calories

These breakfasts stand a much better chance of getting you to lunchtime without the trip to the snack machine.

You don't have to take my word for it. At the VA Medical Center in Minneapolis, 14 men were served either a low-fibre cereal or a high-fibre cereal in the morning. Four hours later they were offered lunch – all they could eat. Each subject filled out a questionnaire before the lunch asking them how hungry they were. Those who ate the high-fibre cereal were less hungry, and they also ate less at lunch than did their low-fibre-cereal counterparts. The fibre sticks with you; you feel full for longer. So you may not need the snack machine, and you might even eat less at lunch.

There is no similar study for a low-carbohydrate version of this breakfast, comparing say, croissants with the omelette and bacon breakfast. In studies, subjects on the low-carb diet ate fewer calories per day than their counterparts on other diets without experiencing excess hunger. The high satiating qualities of proteins is one of the most effective aspects of a low-carb diet.

Eating breakfast even makes you smarter! In several studies published over the past 25 years, when individuals who have had breakfast are given tasks that require concentration and memory, they do better than their unbreakfasted counterparts.

So maybe eating breakfast makes you smarter, and maybe more thin people eat breakfast, but does it help you get thinner and stay thinner? There is research that suggests it does. At Vanderbilt University, 52 women were divided into two groups and put on a 12-week diet. Both were supposed to eat the same number of calories per day, but one group was supposed to eat breakfast and the other was supposed to skip breakfast. Everybody lost weight – an average of 7.75kg (17lb) in 12 weeks – but those who ate breakfast reported less hunger and less impulsive snacking.

And successful dieters are much more likely to eat breakfast than the average person. In America, the National Weight Control Registry, a group of 3,000 men and women who are successful dieters (on average they have lost more than 27kg (4 stone 4lb) and kept it off for more than 6 years) were surveyed about their eating habits, and almost 80 per cent said they ate breakfast every day. Only 4 per cent reported that they never ate breakfast. Statistics on adult eating habits are hard to come by, but in a recent Gallup poll on children, fewer than half said that they ate breakfast. I can only imagine that the rate among adults is even lower.

One last word on breakfast: sumo wrestlers skip breakfast. It's part of their centuries-old tradition of gaining weight. It works for them, and trust me, it can work for you too. So, eat breakfast, but make it worth your while by eating a variety of low-fat, high-fibre foods.

What about skipping other meals? One of the problems when you skip a meal is that you get hungry, and when you get hungry, it is very hard to stop eating when you've had enough. One of the primary predictors of how much someone is going to eat at a given time is how hungry they are when they sit down at the table. If you eat only one meal a day, you give up control of your eating when you finally sit down for that meal, because you're starved.

And being that hungry makes overeating easy. You haven't eaten all day, and the hungrier you are, the faster you tend to eat. You shovel it in, and the mechanisms that are in place to tell you to stop are overwhelmed. By the time your body tells you that you have eaten enough, you have eaten way more than enough.

There is also evidence that being without food causes the stress hormones in your body to get revved up. You don't even have to go all day without eating to get your stress hormones going. In a study published in *The New England Journal of Medicine*, researchers looked at the effect of two types of eating: nibbling and gorging. Men assigned to the nibbling group ate 17 snacks over the course of the day but no big meals. Gorgers ate the more traditional three meals per day. The researchers were mostly interested in seeing if changing how these men ate would change their cholesterol, but they measured other body chemicals as well. Nibbling definitely improved the men's cholesterol, but in addition, the researchers found that the nibblers had much lower levels of the hormone associated with stress.

Not eating is a stress on the body, so it's not really surprising that being hungry would cause a higher level of stress hormone. This is a problem when you are trying to lose weight, because stress makes you fat. That's right. The hormones your body puts out when you are stressed, either because of events in your life or because you haven't eaten, direct your body to stop burning fat. And chronic stress makes you put the fat on in a particular area – your stomach. So by skipping meals, you are actually making yourself fatter, not thinner.

The other problem with eating only one meal per day is that one meal isn't really enough. What happens then is snacking. With many people who eat only one meal per day, that one meal lasts all evening long.

So, how many meals is the right amount? Three, 5, 17? There is some evidence that how many meals is not as important as the day-to-day pattern of eating. Overeating occurs more frequently in those who don't have a regular pattern. A number of analyses indicate that whether you eat 3, 5 or 10 meals or snacks has little direct effect on energy balance. It's not the actual number of meals that is most important, but it's consistency on a daily basis.

In a recent study, researchers found that high day-to-day variation in energy intakes were associated with higher fat and BMI. A degree of regularity and structure to daily eating may also reduce the chances for opportunistic or emotion-driven breakdowns in dietary restraint.

Bottom line: eat breakfast every day, and try to maintain a pattern of eating that keeps you from getting hungry and that you can stick with routinely.

SNACKING AND HUNGER

So is there anything wrong with snacking if you get hungry between meals? No, it is important to eat when you are hungry, not when you are starving. On the other hand, there has been a pretty dramatic increase in the amount of food we consume as snacks versus meals, and this has paralleled our increasing weight. Over the past 25 years, our snacking has increased 200 per cent – that is, the number of calories we take in as snacks – but our intake at mealtime has decreased only a very small amount. In other words, we are eating more snacks in addition to what we already eat.

Snacking can be helpful in weight control by keeping you from getting too hungry between meals. If you get too hungry, you end up eating much more at a meal than you otherwise might. Also, when you are hungry, your ability to avoid food that is appealing but not what you should eat diminishes dramatically.

When you find yourself snacking regularly, ask yourself several questions: first, why are you hungry now? One of the reasons that people get hungry is that the food they ate for their last meal didn't hold them until their next meal. If you have a couple of doughnuts for breakfast, it dramatically increases the chances that you will need a snack before lunch. In a study of 14 men and women who were fed meals containing either high or low fibre content, hunger and the sensation of fullness lasted much, much longer after eating the meals with lots of fibre. Studies on other highly sating foods such as proteins have shown similar results. The meals you eat should contain foods that have high satiating powers to increase the chances that you will only get hungry in time for your next meal. So, the first thing you should question when you find yourself hungry between meals is why breakfast or lunch isn't holding.

Of course, it may not be what you ate for your last meal. Another common reason for getting hungry between meals is that the meal is delayed longer than earlier food can expect to hold you over. If you eat lunch at noon but dinner at 8:00 or 9:00 PM, chances are you are going to get hungry before dinnertime.

Some people prefer to eat more frequently than the traditional three square meals per day. The three-meal eating pattern was forced on us by the demands of the industrial age, which allowed only one break during the workday to maximize productivity. So there is really no reason to consider three meals the magic number. You may be someone who prefers to eat more frequently.

If you like eating more frequently, that's fine, but, of course, you need to plan for this. Chances are that there is nothing in a snack machine that is good for you to eat. In general, the ideal snack should have some carbohydrate component to fill you up and some protein component to make it last. An apple with a small chunk of cheese is one obvious snack, a small container of yoghurt is another. A handful of nuts is a good snack for those of you who are trying to limit carbohydrate intake. Probably none of these (except maybe the nuts) are going to be available at your local vending machine. So, if you are a snacker, take a snack with you to work or wherever you go. If you leave your snacking choices to the marketplace, you will end up taking in much more food than you need, and that will simply increase your food intake for the day. Who needs that?

This assumes that the reason you are snacking is because you are hungry. That's not always the case. People often snack for other reasons. Maybe you are bored or stressed. Or, and this is very common, maybe you have come to expect to snack when you engage in a particular activity – like watching television – and so the trigger to eat isn't hunger but something else. Here is what makes that snacking different from snacking when you are hungry: snacking when you are hungry helps you eat less when you sit down to your next meal. Eating when you are not hungry doesn't. In fact, your body doesn't register these snacks as food at all. They just go in, and the calorie meter in our brains that tries to make sure we eat about the same amount every day doesn't even register these calories. They just end up as extra.

When you find yourself cruising for a snack, first ask yourself, 'Am I hungry, or is this something else?' When you are hungry, figure out why, and then go get yourself a snack you can work consistently into your everyday routine. If you are not hungry, figure out what the trigger is, and try to find some other activity to satisfy your need. I know: it's not easy! When you are stressed or upset, you may not even want to think about the big picture, but it's important.

You have to remember that your eating patterns are with you until you change them. They will not change on their own.

If stress is an obvious trigger for you, then you have to deal with it more creatively. Once you do that, you have a much better chance of making a lasting change in the way you eat, even after you're at your ideal level.

Bottom line: between-meal hunger may be due to meals of poorly satiating foods. Other possibilities include 'hunger' due to emotional causes or a preference for more frequent meals. Make sure you eat meals that will last, and if you still want snacks, take them with you.

EMOTIONAL EATING

If you scored 15 or more on the Emotional Eating section of the questionnaire, you have a tendency to eat when you aren't hungry. Or you may be using food to feed your spirit rather than your stomach, and that can add quite a bit of weight. While the behaviours are the same

– eating when you are not hungry – this section covers two very different phenomena: emotional eating and habitual eating. Let's start with emotional eating, then we'll talk about what I call mindless eating.

Feelings can make people eat. I'm not talking about feeling hunger, I'm talking about other kinds of feelings – emotions. Many of us eat in response to feelings – often bad feelings.

Barbara, a 35-year-old divorced mother of two, finds herself in her office kitchen eating biscuits whenever she gets angry or annoyed at a colleague. Just the act of putting that biscuit in her mouth, she says, helps her get her thoughts together and figure out how to deal with her anger.

Janet, a 32-year-old legal assistant to a high-powered lawyer, rewards herself with a chunk of dark chocolate after a stressful day at the office. She feels like she 'deserves' it.

Kathy, an energetic 36-year-old social worker and divorced mother of two teenage boys, comforts herself late at night with a big bowl of ice cream when her loneliness feels unbearable. She takes care of her clients, her family and her friends, but at the end of the day she feels too drained to take care of herself. That's when the ice cream really helps.

Matt, a successful 40-year-old businessman, craves Skittles before going to an important deal. Chewing these fruity bits on the way to the meeting gives him an outlet for the excitement he feels when 'going in for the kill'.

All of these people came to me for help in finding a diet that would allow them to take charge of their weight. Turning to food when confronted with overwhelming emotion seems as natural and inevitable to them – and to many of us – as scratching an itch or yawning with fatigue.

In order to understand that link, and ultimately break it, we have to understand the nature of stress and our bodies. In each instance, the desire for food comes in the face of overwhelming stress. It is a natural response – one programmed into us at a very primitive level, but one that leads to overeating, weight gain and, ultimately, unhappiness.

Let's talk about stress – what it is and what it does to us. Our bodies' reaction to stress is something we share with most, if not all, species in the animal kingdom. We perceive a threat to our well-being – a big, hungry animal or a mugger – and immediately our bodies change in order to respond to that threat: our hearts start to beat faster, we breathe faster, our eyes dilate, we stop digesting our food so that the blood that had been going to the gastrointestinal tract can go to our muscles. Thinking is slower, but reflex or gut responses are quicker. At the chemical level, we get a rush of adrenaline as well as another type of stress-response hormone: cortisol. All of these changes, known in school biology terms as the fight-or-flight response, put us in peak form to cope with this life-threatening event.

That response worked great on the African savannah – in fact, without it we most certainly wouldn't have survived. But here in modern civilization it's not quite as useful. Sure, it's still helpful when the stressful event is something that requires either fight or flight – like a mugger in a dark alley – but most of our most stressful events in modern life are not direct threats to life and limb.

Modern life attacks us with emotional threats and stressors. But just because our physical being isn't threatened doesn't mean those stressors aren't important or painful. We all go through major life stresses that don't lay a hand on us: the death of someone we love, divorce, getting fired. And there are other stressors that affect us on a more regular basis: missing a plane, having an argument, being late, meeting deadlines. In many people these daily stresses also trigger that same life-or-death reaction: adrenaline and cortisol start flowing; blood pressure, heart rate and respiratory rate go up; and we're physically ready to fight off the attackers. Not very helpful in dealing with these kinds of stressors. And it's that response you are fighting when you tell yourself (on your good days, anyway), 'Okay, take a deep breath. Calm down and deal with it.'

Fight-or-flight is not well-suited to the stresses we meet in our everyday lives. And chronic exposure to the stress response can make us fat and unhealthy. Over the past 20 years, researchers around the world have been interested in the effects of stress on health. In multiple studies, it has been shown that excessive and sustained cortisol are associated with depression, high blood pressure, osteoporosis, a suppressed immune system and metabolic syndrome, along with higher rates of atherosclerosis and heart disease.

The physiology of this is still being worked out, but here's what we know so far: adrenaline is the chemical that gets our hearts and lungs going and sends our blood pressure up. Cortisol has the job of finding the fuel to keep things running. Cortisol calls up the glucose we have stored in our livers and sends it to our brains, our hearts, our lungs and our muscles to help us fight off an attacker or take off running. After the initial response to the stress is over, the adrenaline recedes, but the cortisol stays on to try to get things back to normal.

One of the things that cortisol does is to get us to eat; that way we can replace the glucose and fat that was liberated. Again, it worked well on the savannahs, but in response to deadlines and daily stress, we don't actually use that much of the freed fuel; most of it just ends up back in storage. Unfortunately, cortisol doesn't know that. It just goes about its job to get us to eat and we do, willingly. (The physiology of this is beautifully described in *Fight Fat after Forty*, by Dr Pamela Peeke, one of the scientists involved in this groundbreaking research. If you want to know more about how stress affects us, I highly recommend this book.)

We have already seen that, under stress, people head for sweets and fats and consume extra calories. It's not just humans who eat this way under stress. In a series of experiments, rats who were stressed by having a researcher pinch their tails were noted to eat even when they had just finished a meal and were probably not hungry. And when they ate, they preferred sweet and fatty rat food over their normal food.

There may be a biological reason for this preference for high-fat foods during stress: there is good evidence that these intrinsically appealing foods stimulate the brain's built-in reward system, the release of endorphins, so that you actually do feel better when you eat them. In addition, high-fat foods might be more easily eaten and digested when digestive-tract activity is suppressed by stress.

So now you know: stress makes you eat, and when you are stressed, you prefer calorie-dense, sweet foods. I suspect that this is not a big surprise to many of you. It's not much of a surprise to most of my patients. Still, it's nice to know that it's not just you or your lack of willpower. It's a natural response to the world we live in.

On the other hand, I'm certainly not advising you to just accept that and live with it. If stress is making you eat, you have to figure out a way to reduce your stress where possible and give yourself a replacement stress-reducer for unavoidable pressure.

What can you do to reduce stress? First of all, I tell my patients that they have to learn how to say no. The only way to reduce your stress is to make more room for yourself in your life. Your needs – physical and mental – have to be put higher on your priority list. This means that other people will not always think you are perfect. Trying to be perfect for others is one of the key causes of stress in this world. You need to take care of yourself, and sometimes that means that you take care of others less.

And with the extra time you will have once you start saying no to others' needs, you need to start doing things for yourself. They ought to be things that will help you combat the ravages of the stress you just can't avoid. Exercise has been shown to help; meditation helps; eating in a way that is good for you helps. Just about anything you can do to make your life better will help you to better deal with the stress the world forces on us.

There are stresses that can't be avoided, those that are part of your everyday life. Deadlines, for example, are common stressors; travel is another stressor that frequently gets that adrenaline and cortisol going. What can you do about these? When you know you have a stressful day or week before you, you should plan for it. Try to get your exercise in early. Take your meals with you. Try to get a good night's sleep. You need to plan for these events so that they don't take their usual toll on you and your waistline.

Bottom line: when you feel that stress-induced need to feed, go for a walk, go shopping, do something that will really make you feel good. Don't just eat, because you know in the long run it doesn't help.

HABITUAL EATING

There are lots of reasons to eat besides being hungry or feeling upset. For example, you go out to dinner and to the movies. You buy a bag of popcorn even though you just ate. Despite the fact that you're not hungry, it tastes good and feels right. In fact, it's hard to imagine going to the movies and not eating popcorn. This is an example of eating that's triggered by something other than the experience of hunger. In this case, it is triggered by habit. You always get popcorn when you go to the movies, so even when you are not hungry, you get popcorn. If you don't, it feels odd. That's because you've made a link between these two activities, so that whenever you do the one, you want to do the other. It's one of the many ways we take in calories without even noticing.

What if you got a medium bag of popcorn with butter and a medium cola? These days that seems like a modest movie-viewing purchase. The popcorn is 500 calories (only 300 without the butter) and a 360ml (12fl-oz) cola is around 145 calories. Without really thinking about it, you've consumed 645 calories. And you weren't even hungry!

Another common opportunity for eating without hunger is watching television. This may be the number one eating-activity pairing. It is certainly the one most solidly linked to obesity. In a recent study published in *JAMA*, researchers at Harvard followed more than 50,000 women over 6 years who were either normal weight or somewhat over the average weight. During that time, 3,800 women, just under 8 per cent of them, became very overweight. When those women were compared to women who were similar in BMI, exercise level, smoking status and diet, the primary difference between the women who gained a lot of weight and those who didn't was television. And the more television they watched, the greater their risk of getting fat.

You might think that the weight gain was just from inactivity and not specific to television, but when these researchers compared having a sedentary job or the amount of time spent reading or playing board games, television watching created a much bigger risk for weight gain.

Why is that? One theory is that watching television makes you eat. Food advertising on television is ubiquitous – in a study done in America more than 10 years ago, researchers noted a commercial for food every 4 minutes. Moreover, more than 60 per cent of these commercials were for high-fat, low-nutritional-value foods.

Since these women were bombarded with these ads for bad foods, the thought was that they were more likely to eat them. And, in fact, the women in this study did report eating more calories per day with a higher intake of high-fat, low-nutritional-value foods. There have been studies showing similar associations between watching TV and higher food intake in men and children too.

Could not watching television, then, be a weight-reduction

strategy? Researchers in California recently showed that by reducing the amount of television children watched as well as the frequency of eating in front of the television, overweight children lost weight. It worked for them, so chances are, if you're a big-time TV watcher, it will work for you.

TV might be our worst problem, but it's not the only one. Some people read, others drive. One patient of mine has a hard time talking on the phone if she's not nibbling on 'a little something'. If you eat a snack because you are hungry, when you get to the next meal, you are less hungry, so you eat less. But when you eat even though you aren't hungry, it doesn't change how much you eat at your next meal. So this snack that you are not even hungry for just adds that many more calories to what you eat in a day, without even addressing the real issue – the real danger in trying to lose weight – hunger.

Moreover, when you eat while you are doing something else, you tend to eat more. This is true even if you are hungry. Reading the paper, talking on the phone, driving – these activities distract you from your bodies' cues that you have had enough to eat. In a series of experiments in France, researchers watched 40 normal-weight women as they ate under different conditions. One meal they ate alone, with no distractions; at another meal, each ate listening to a tape of a detective story, and then finally, they ate together in groups of four. For all the women, eating while distracted, that is while listening to the story on tape, caused them to eat more – much more – than when they were eating alone or eating in a group.

Bottom line: don't eat when you're not hungry – those calories taken in are the real empty ones. And when you are hungry, don't eat while you are doing something else.

CHAPTER 14

LIFESTYLE

EATING OUT

If you have a score of 20 or higher in the Eating Out section, then eating away from home is likely to be a factor in your difficulty in losing weight or maintaining your weight loss.

Just 25 years ago, the majority of the food we ate was eaten at home. Now, in some age groups, particularly amongst 18 to 34 year olds, almost half the food we eat is eaten out. We are now twice as likely to eat at a restaurant or fast-food joint as we used to be (the average is two meals a week).

Working life forces some of this change on us, whether we like it or not. Few of us live close enough to work to actually go home for lunch, or sometimes even for supper. And often, in this climate of pressure for higher productivity, mealtime is one of the rare occasions we have to relax and enjoy time with our colleagues and friends at work. So we can find ourselves going out to lunch virtually every day or, at the other end of the spectrum, trying to skip lunch. It seems as though our work schedules are conspiring to make us fat.

In fact, there is some evidence that they are. In a recent study from Japan, where obesity is growing almost as fast as it is in America, researchers followed a large group of workers over a period of 3 years. There was a good correlation between the number of overtime hours worked and weight. The more they worked, the fatter these mostly male workers became. The researchers speculated that it was a combination of a change in eating habits (eating more meals at work rather than at home) and less time in which to exercise. The same study done in the US or the UK would, I suspect, reveal the same. Obviously, when eating at home, we have much more control over what we eat than we do when we eat out.

It's not just where we eat that has changed. What we eat when we do eat out has also changed dramatically – in size. When you look at the food pyramid or any of the dietary recommendations put out by nutrition agencies, amounts of food are usually described by number of servings. According to the original food pyramid, we are supposed to eat five to seven servings of grains, breads or pasta per day. We're not told what that serving size should be. A serving is a serving is a serving – right? No. These guidelines are based on what the average serving size was when these guidelines were developed in the 1980s. What a difference 20 years has made!

A recent American study compared current serving sizes of commonly consumed foods that could be bought when eating out today with those used in the food pyramid and on food labels. The difference was mind boggling.

Say someone had a bagel for breakfast. The recommended serving size is 60g (2oz), but the bagel available in some supermarkets is 125g (4½oz) – more than twice the bagel it used to be. If you go for a muffin, the recommended serving size is also 60g (2oz). The average – this is the *average*, not the biggest – was more than three times that size, and some muffins were six times that size! That means that with one muffin, you have eaten all the grains and breads you are supposed to eat for the rest of the day! It would be okay if you knew that and adjusted for it, but who knew?

Let's move on to lunch. Say you had a hamburger; you're watching your weight, so you pass on the fries. The recommended weight of your burger and your bun together should be 115g (4oz). Remember, though this seems small to you now, these sizes were based on the average size of the portion back in the 1980s, when the pyramid was designed. The current fast-food burger-bun combo is larger as well, at around 170g (6oz). However, at some American chain restaurant, that burger-bun combo could be *twice* the size of the pyramid portion, at 250g (9oz). That's very close to the maximum daily amount of meat recommended on the food pyramid.

Okay, how about supper? You had a burger for lunch, so you figure you'll eat light for dinner. How about some pasta? At a chain restaurant, the average serving of pasta can be as much as four times larger than the recommended allowance for a serving of pasta.

The US undoubtedly leads the way on this front so it's little surprise that average calorie intake there has increased by 600 calories a day in the past 30 years – 600 calories a day! You do the maths: there are 3,500 calories in 455g (1lb) of fat. Increasing your calorie count by 600 calories per day means that you put on an average of 455g (1lb) every 6 days! No wonder that over the past 20 years the percentage of Americans who are overweight has doubled.

Americans, and increasingly Britons, have recognized this change in portion size and welcomed it – although I suspect they didn't really understand what it meant to the real bottom line, the waistline. You can't accuse American restaurant chains of not responding to consumer demand. They heard, and they were more than happy to oblige with huge servings of bad food.

The same supersizing trend has moved into vending machines too. Look at chocolate bars and packets of crisps. They just keep getting bigger and bigger.

Let me remind you: portion size is learned. How do we know this? The first evidence came from experiments on rats. In laboratories rats were given as much rat food as they wanted. Once this portion size was determined, the rats were fed that amount daily. After a week or so of this, the portion size was increased.

At first, the rats continued to eat the same amount of food, leaving the excess untouched. But after several days, the rats started eating the excess. When allowed to eat freely in an unrestricted fashion, as they had been originally, they ate this bigger portion but no more. They had learned a new portion size, which they then expected to eat at each meal.

We behave the same way as lab rats. Barbara Rolls, PhD, decided to check this portion theory out. She recruited a group of adults and had them eat several meals. Before each meal, each person was asked to rate his hunger. Then they were served a meal. What the participants didn't know was that with each meal they were being served larger and larger portions. Despite having the same amount of hunger, these volunteers ate the larger portions. They learned a new portion size.

This is not just a laboratory phenomenon either. The same thing has happened here in the real world as well. Greg Critser, in his book, *Fat Land*, suggests that Americans (and increasingly Britons) have been inside a giant portion laboratory since fast-food franchises started selling more (food) for less (money) 15 years ago. It all started with Taco Bell. Some of their market research suggested that the reason people came back to the their restaurants over and over and over again was not because of taste or quality but because of value and savings. So, the Taco Bell head honcho took a risk: what if he made the food an even bigger bargain? Would customers come back even more frequently?

They cut their prices and held their collective breath. The word went out and . . . business boomed. But what was really amazing – even to the executive at Taco Bell – the people who came didn't end up spending less money. Instead, they bought more food. Like the rats, when presented with more food (for the same amount of money), we might have balked initially, but in no time we ate it, enjoyed it, and finally insisted on it.

In the few short years since Taco Bell made this remarkable discovery, everybody's got in on the act. Value meals – under one name or the other – are ubiquitous. And it's not just in fast-food joints either. Everywhere you go, food has been supersized. Even the finest restaurants now heap food onto our plates. Name a food and the chances are that over the past decade the serving size has grown. Soft drinks are bigger; doughnuts are bigger; chocolate bars are bigger; a slice of pizza is bigger; even salads are bigger.

No matter what type of diet you end up on, managing your weight requires that you scale down your portion sizes. If big portions can be learned, so can small portions. The problem is that you will be doing this on your own. Don't expect restaurants and vending machines to reduce the size of their portions. It's been way too profitable for them to reverse the trend.

Larger portion sizes in foods we eat away from home have undoubtedly contributed to our expanding waistlines, but the world we live in often makes it difficult not to eat out. So what's your average working person to do?

There are some tricks to eating out that may make it easier for you. There's no magic here, just common sense.

1. Take your lunch and snacks to work with you. When you are trying to lose weight, it's easier to control both what you eat and how much of it you eat when you make it yourself.

2. If you eat your lunch at your desk, use the extra time that you would have spent had you gone out to lunch by taking a brisk walk or exercising with your friends.

3. If you have to eat a meal out, take snacks to work so that when you do go out for lunch or supper, you're not so hungry that you inhale the bread as soon as you sit down.

4. Order one or two appetizers rather than a main course. The appetizers come more quickly, so you don't have to wait as long to eat. You'll be surprised at how much they fill you up. Appetizers have also grown, and often, what is now considered an appetizer used to be a whole serving.

5. Order a half size or appetizer size of a pasta or other main dish. If the restaurant doesn't do that, ask the server to bring you only half and pack the rest up for you to take home, or split the dish with a friend.

6. Send away the bread before it even lands on the table.

7. Don't hesitate to tell the server how you would like your food prepared. If you want it grilled rather than fried or with the sauce on the side, ask for it that way. A restaurant would rather let you 'have it your way' and come back again than not.

8. Find the restaurants in your area that serve foods that you can eat on your diet. A fat-counting diet is the hardest to pursue when eating out, because restaurants add fats to just about everything to improve flavour and appearance.

9. Get all sauces served on the side.

10. Eat the foods that you'll feel good about eating first. Save the higher-calorie foods for last. When you get a steak and salad, eat the salad first.

11. Avoid drinking an alcoholic beverage before your meal, and limit your alcohol consumption during a meal.

12. When you know you are going to be dining out, allow for the extra calories you will undoubtedly consume by being selective in what you eat before and after your restaurant meal.

13. When you overeat, forgive yourself and get back on the diet – before you add insult to injury by eating dessert too.

One last point: many of my patients have told me that when they go out to eat with their friends and order just an appetizer or a salad, they worry that their friends perceive this as an assault on their eating habits, since they are ordering the usual big lunch. I suspect that this is true some of the time. But the world we live in is pushing us down the path to obesity. If you want to get off that path, it's going to make you different. Here's your choice: you can continue with them on their path and end up with the same weight problems as your friends, or you can find your own way to the weight you want.

Sometimes others may feel that the choices you make for yourself imply a criticism about them. It's not that. You know that as well as I do. Their feelings are a projection of their own concerns about their weight. They have to make their own choices. You must be free to make yours.

DAILY ACTIVITY

A score of 45 or less in the Daily Activity part of the questionnaire indicates that your activity level is contributing to your difficulty in maintaining the weight you want.

In the UK, levels of physical activity are below the European average and research suggests a third of the population are mostly sedentary. That's what they admit to. Here's what we know about physical activity: it makes you feel better and live longer, it helps you lose weight and maintain weight loss once you've achieved your ideal weight, and you don't have to exercise to get the benefits that physical activity has to offer. If physical activity isn't exercise, what is it? Basically, it's anything you do that requires you to move. Many of us live our lives in an environment that only asks us to walk from the house to the car, then a few steps from the car to the office, and spend the rest of the day sitting, except for a few steps to the bathroom and the canteen and then back to the car.

Physical activity is anything we do that is more than that. Walking down the hall to communicate with a colleague rather than just sending a quick e-mail. Parking in the most distant parking space to add a brisk walk to each end of your day. Walking the kids to school rather than driving. A recent study showed that people who live in an urban setting tend to be thinner than those who live in the suburbs. Why is that? Because urbanites have to walk more than their suburban counterparts.

Researchers in the 1990s looked at physical activity and saw that much of the cardiovascular benefit accrued even when the activity was not vigorous and didn't last half an hour. And, of course, any activity will burn calories.

A study done a few years ago compared the weight-loss benefit of increasing daily activity versus adding an exercise regime in response to the traditional recommendation to exercise more. Several thousand sedentary, overweight adults were divided into two groups. Both groups were instructed to follow a weight-reduction diet, and one group was instructed to exercise for 30 minutes per day. The other was counselled to increase their everyday activity by walking up stairs, parking a couple of streets from work, and standing rather than sitting.

Initially, the group instructed to exercise lost more weight, but after 2 years the two groups had evened out. In fact, more people in the activity group were getting 30 minutes of exercise at least three times per week than in the exercise group. Moreover, in both groups, the individuals who were more active reported more weight loss and feeling better overall.

So even if you hate the gym, can't stand sweating, wouldn't work out if your life depended on it, you can increase the amount of activity in your life and reap many of the benefits of exercising without actually having to do it.

What can you do?

1. Take the stairs rather than the lift. Walking up one flight of stairs can burn off 10 calories. You might think that's not very much, but if you did a couple of flights every day, it would soon add up.

2. Don't drive all the way to work. Park a couple of streets away and walk the difference. If you walk one-fifth of a mile, you burn off 20 to 25 calories. Do it both ways and you're making a difference.

3. Try standing while you watch television. Standing for an hour can burn 100 calories. Pacing can also help. You burn off a calorie with each 15 steps taken.

4. If you have a sit-down job, think up reasons to get up and walk. Rather than e-mail a colleague, walk over to his office and see him. Rather than send something by internal mail, take it yourself.

5. Take a short walk every day before lunch. It will make your lunch taste better, and a brisk 15- to 20-minute walk can burn off 100 calories.

6. Use businesses that are relatively close to your home or office, and walk there when you do errands instead of driving there.

7. Keep track of your activity. Anything you do that has you moving can be counted as activity. On the opposite page is a list of activities and the calories you burn doing them for just 10 minutes. See if you can increase the calories you burn by just a few calories per day.

CALORIES BURNED IN EVERYDAY ACTIVITIES

Activity	Calories Burned in 10 Minutes Body weight: 57kg (125lb)	Calories Burned in 10 Minutes Body weight: 80kg (175lb)
Carpentry	32	44
Chopping wood	60	84
Cycling (5.5 mph)	42	58
Dancing (moderate)	35	48
Dressing or washing	26	37
House painting	29	40
Light gardening	30	42
Light office work	25	34
Making beds	32	46
Mowing the lawn (using power mower)	34	47
Preparing food	32	46
Shovelling snow	65	90
Sitting (watching TV)	10	14
Sitting and talking	15	21
Sleeping	10	14
Standing	12	15
Standing (light activity)	20	28
Table tennis	32	45
Walking (2 mph)	29	40
Walking (4 mph)	52	72
Walking down stairs	56	78
Walking up stairs	146	202
Washing floors	35	48
Weeding	49	68

EXERCISE

If you have a score of more than 10 in the Exercise section of the questionnaire, then you probably are having some difficulty getting yourself to work out. Here's the problem with that: without exercise, you dramatically reduce the likelihood that you will be able to maintain your weight loss. It's as simple as that.

Let me remind you of the good that exercise provides.

1. It burns off calories, which allows you to eat a few more goodies than you would be able to without exercise.
2. It reduces stress and improves symptoms of depression.
3. It decreases mortality.
4. It makes your body feel better.
5. It makes your body look better.
6. It reduces your appetite (in the long run).
7. It makes you think more clearly.
8. Exercise will really increase your metabolism and allow you to burn off more calories even when you sleep.

So what are the barriers to exercise? They are as many and diverse as we are. While how much we eat has increased, the amount of activity in our lives has decreased. Although the vast majority of us describe ourselves as sedentary, I would argue that we are not sedentary because we are lazy. We were not built to be sedentary, but the way our world is structured right now makes it hard not to be. You have to work in order to restore a natural level of activity to life.

A woman now spends 400 calories less in a single day's activity than a woman at the start of the 20th century. We are not hauling water or scrubbing floors on our knees or bringing in wood to keep the home fires burning. And thank God. Believe me, I am not advocating a return to earlier times. But what this means is that activity, the natural exercise we are all designed for, has been taken out of the realm of everyday life and now has to be put back intentionally.

That can feel fake and somewhat silly. When you are busy, it can seem dopey to walk to the shops or to cycle to work, when it's just faster and more efficient to drive. And taking the stairs rather than the lift can often appear an odd choice, especially since the stairs are frequently dark and dirty and hard to find. Then, after working a full day and taking care of everyone at home, we are expected to choose to spend our rare free time exercising? It seems an unreasonable choice to many, and so most people are sedentary.

And yet, the physical, mental and psychological benefits of exercise are undeniable. The first reason I get from my patients as to why they are not exercising is that they don't have time. And many of my patients have families, which means that they work at their job and then come home and work that second unpaid job. There is no doubt that these people are very busy.

The second reason offered by most of my patients is that they don't like to exercise. I suspect that is really the reason that most of us don't exercise. We just haven't found a way to do it that feels good and is enjoyable. But we must. I can't promise you that you will achieve your ideal weight. I can't promise you that you will have the body you so long for. But here is a promise I feel 100 per cent comfortable making: if you exercise, you will feel better. Period.

Our bodies are designed to move, even when they are out of shape and overweight. If you move, your body will feel better and so will the rest of you. The trick, I think, is to find some way to move that suits you that you can incorporate into your everyday life.

First, let's think about what you don't like about exercise. Well, there's the whole time thing: it's just one more thing that you have to incorporate into an already busy life. That's true. But who takes care of the caretaker? If you spend your days taking care of other you need to make time and space for yourself in order to keep up that caretaking.

The actress and comedienne Lily Tomlin said something really wise in one of her monologues: 'For fast-acting relief, try slowing down.' Slow down; take some time for yourself, even if it means doing less for others. One of the reasons my patients don't do this is because they want others to think that they are perfect: perfectly competent and capable; perfectly able to take care of everything. The only one they can stint on, if that is their goal, is themselves. And they do it. Frequently. So, make time for yourself. You make time for others. Are you a morning person? Get up half an hour earlier and use that time to exercise. Are you a night owl? Stay up a little later and use the extra time to exercise.

Another barrier to exercise is lack of experience. Many people have never exercised, or at least not in a long, long time. Because it's been so long, they don't remember the good feeling they got after exercising. Trust me – it's there.

The fear of not being good at something is another hurdle. We're out of the habit of learning new things, many of us. We're uneasy at the prospect of looking like a beginner. So, why not start by doing something you already know how to do? The most popular exercise is walking, and that's a perfect place to start. You don't need any special equipment and you don't need to be fit.

Some people don't want to be seen exercising. They are embarrassed about their bodies or their physical skills. Do something you can do at home. Get an exercise video and work out along with that. Get a treadmill. Get an exercise bike. Do your exercises in a pleasant environment, and make an effort to maximize the pleasure you get from them. Do it in front of the TV set. Or listen to books on tape or to music. Try to make it fun.

Starting to exercise takes a certain amount of what chemistry calls 'activation energy'. It takes more energy to get started, but once you do, it's not nearly as hard to continue. Remember that when you are lying in bed trying to think of good reasons not to get up and out.

Finally, I think many of my patients have very little experience with the huge variety available in exercise. They have tried running or walking or cycling and didn't like it, so their conclusion is that they don't like exercise. Keep trying. Don't be afraid to try different exercises. How about yoga? Or tai chi? Pilates? Dance workouts? Be creative. Find something you like and stick with it.

When you start off, start slow and low. If you haven't really exercised in quite a long time, you can start by doing just 10 minutes. After a few weeks, add another 10 minutes. It doesn't have to be 20 minutes at a stretch; 10 and 10 work just as well.

And you don't have to exercise until you 'feel the burn'. The way you gauge the effort you are expending is to measure your pulse. The faster your heart is beating, the harder you are working. But the best way to burn fat is not by working the hardest – the hardest work is good for your heart. But the best speed to burn off fat is much lower, and that's good news to many of us.

Here's how to determine your target heart rate. For starters, get a calculator; you'll need it.

To calculate the rate for burning fat, subtract your age from 220:

$$220 - \underline{\qquad} = \underline{\qquad}$$

Multiply that by 0.65:

$$\underline{\qquad} \times 0.65 = \underline{\qquad} \text{ beats per minute}$$

That number is your target heart rate when you want to burn fat. For a cardiovascular workout, again subtract your age from 220:

$$220 - \underline{\qquad} = \underline{\qquad}$$

This time multiply that number by 0.85:

$$\underline{\qquad} \times 0.85 = \underline{\qquad} \text{ beats per minute}$$

I usually check my pulse at my carotid artery. It is located just under the angle of your jaw on your neck. It's not easy to miss. I count for 10 seconds and then multiply that number by 6 to get the beats per minute.

Many of my patients who finally fell in love with exercise started by exercising with a friend. It tends to keep you honest and motivated. You and your buddy can take turns being the lazy one and the energetic one. And it's a great way to make exercise a little more fun, and that's particularly important at the beginning.

After you have started walking, cycling, swimming, or whatever you decide works for you, you need to consider adding weight lifting, or resistance training, to the programme. Weight lifting builds muscle better than any other activity. The more muscle you have, the higher your metabolism. The higher your metabolism, the more calories you burn in your sleep.

In weight or resistance training, how you do it – form – is the most important thing. So, consider getting a few lessons from a weight trainer in your area. You don't have to join a gym; you can do this stuff at home, but you need to do it correctly.

How much exercise do you need? Less than you might think. The official recommendation is 30 minutes a day for most days of the week. If you aim at 150 minutes per week, I think you'll find that's sufficient.

Pay attention to your body and try to have fun. Here's my promise again. If you exercise, you *will* feel better.

AFTERWORD

◆

'To eat is a necessity, but to eat intelligently is an art.'
— FRANCOIS LA ROCHEFOUCAULD, MAXIMS 1665

The goal of this book has been to teach you the art of eating intelligently. Only by eating wisely will we be able to manage our weight in a world that eagerly and aggressively seeks to fatten us up. To achieve this wisdom, we need to combine what science has to teach us about eating and exercise with what we know about ourselves. Of these two, I would say that self-knowledge is the most important. Nevertheless, in this book I have aspired to provide you with the tools to acquire both.

The questionnaire will help you understand the hows and whys of the ways you eat. This knowledge will help you to identify the characteristics of your diet – the one you developed over your lifetime of eating – and with that knowledge you can begin to understand what can be changed and what cannot. The information about the nutrition and physiology of eating will guide you to making choices about the diet and lifestyle you need to stay healthy and fit for the rest of your life.

Of course, the questionnaire and the research on nutrition and diet provide a snapshot of two very dynamic processes. Inevitably both will change over time. It's easiest to see in the context of your own life: you get a new job, and – boom – you're spending lots more time at work. It's suddenly hard to find time to exercise (again). Your diet seems to spin out of control (again) as you eat your way through lunch after lunch with new colleagues and contacts. Or maybe you have a baby and not only do you have to lose weight (again), your life is suddenly a lot more complicated.

Nor does it take life-altering events like these to change the choices you've made about diet and exercise. What happens if you get injured while running? What happens if your treadmill breaks or your gym goes out of business? All of these events will require you to go back and revisit some of the same issues you're dealing with now. Your diet and lifestyle are constantly changing. You need to take charge of those changes and make sure they work for you and your goals. My aim has been to help you recognize patterns in how you eat and live so you can use that understanding to manage your weight. Knowing not only what you eat and do but *why* you do them will help you make choices you can live with.

The science of diet will change too, no doubt. We are at the threshold of a very exciting time in this field. Research scientists and doctors are flocking to this growing area of inquiry. The future will bring new discoveries about how the foods and drugs we put into our bodies work in combination with the genes passed on to us by our parents, in the world we have to live in. These discoveries should make it easier for us to understand how our choices affect us, now and in the future.

In the meantime, however, I have tried to give you enough information so that when your life changes, you'll understand how you can adapt to those changes. This book, I hope, will be your toolbox when life changes necessitate lifestyle change.

Finally, you may be wondering, why is all this necessary? Until very recently we didn't need books telling us how to eat and live in order to be healthy. Why now? We are facing a world that has changed in a very fundamental way. Never before has a single population had access to so much food in so much variety and at such a small cost. And never before has the livin' been quite so easy for so many of us.

Too much of our available abundance consists of high-calorie foods that make us fat without necessarily making us full. Agribusiness has been extremely successful: we grow a quantity and variety of foods that would have been unimaginable even 50 years ago.

Because of that incredible success, the overfeeding of the West may well have been unavoidable, at least from a business point of view. Companies that make and sell food, like companies that make and sell just about anything – computers, DVD players, trainers – prosper by selling us more. The problem is that their market is not growing, at least not fast enough. Innovations in agribusiness have allowed food producers in America to make available 3,800 calories per person per day, 700 more than was produced just 30 years ago. In order to maintain profits and continued growth, food companies set out to do what any business would do: persuade each of us to buy – and eat – more, a lot more. And we have.

In supermarkets, on the road, on television, the message is clear and practically continuous: Eat! Eat! Eat! Our bodies were built to withstand the stresses of starvation. In confronting this new stress, the stress of overabundance, we are naked and virtually defenceless, evolutionarily speaking. When the invitation to eat and eat and eat is extended, genetically we are programmed to say yes, yes, yes.

We need to develop strategies to navigate through this new and very different threat. In the distant past, this was the job of genes. More recently, culture has helped us choose the foods that made us survive. But those defences have been outpaced by the rapid changes that mark this time in our history. They may catch up, but genes exert their influence over millennia, and culture over centuries. So we have to figure out our own strategy right now if we want to retain control over our health and well-being. And the only tool we have is education and a willingness to take charge of the way we live and eat.

We are not helpless creatures facing a dangerous world over which we have no control. The choices we make in the marketplace will be heard and felt. Governments and industry can respond to the demands of their constituents and customers. There is a growing movement to change the toxic environment that has pushed America and Britain to become some of the fattest nations in the world. But that kind of change takes time, too, and many of us just can't wait.

The world we live in makes eating intelligently a necessity as well as an art. Making the choices that are right for each of us is our best hope of shaping the lives and bodies we want. This book, I hope, will make that difficult goal just a little easier.

REFERENCES

I reviewed hundreds of articles and books in the writing of this book. Below I have listed books and resources that I depended on throughout the process.

Bellisle, France. 'Cognitive Restraint Can Be Offset by Distraction, Leading to Increased Meal Intake in Women.' *American Journal of Clinical Nutrition* 74 (August 2001): 197–200.

Berne, R. M., and M. N. Levy. *The Principles of Physiology.* St Louis: The CV Mosby Company, 1990.

Bravata, D. M., et al. 'Efficacy and Safety of Low Carbohydrate Diets.' *JAMA* 289, no. 17 (2003): 1837–50.

Davy, Brenda M., and Christopher L. Melby. 'The Effect of Fiber-Rich Carbohydrates on Features of Syndrome X'; Review. *Journal of the American Dietetic Association* 103, no. 1 (2003): 86.

Duffy, V. B., and L. M. Bartoshuk. 'Food Acceptance and Genetic Variation in Taste.' *Journal of the American Dietetic Association* 100, no. 6 (2000): 647–55.

Foster, G. D., et al. 'A Controlled Comparison of Three Very-Low-Calorie Diets: Effects on Weight, Body Composition, and Symptoms.' *American Journal of Clinical Nutrition* 55 (April 1992): 811–17.

Gautier, J. F., et al. 'Effect of Satiation on Brain Activity in Obese and Lean Women.' *Obesity Research* 9 (2001): 729–30.

Goldstein, D. B. 'Pharmacogenetics in the Laboratory and the Clinic.' *New England Journal of Medicine* 348, no. 6 (2003): 553–56.

Hammer, R. L., et al. 'Calorie-Restricted Low-Fat Diet and Exercise in Obese Women.' *American Journal of Clinical Nutrition* 49 (January 1989): 77–85.

Heini, A. F., et al. 'Relationship between Hunger-Satiety Feelings and Various Metabolic Parameters in Women with Obesity during Controlled Weight Loss.' *Obesity Research* 6 (1998): 225–30.

Heitmann, B. L., et al. 'Dietary Underreporting by Obese Individuals – Is It Specific or Nonspecific?' *British Medical Journal* 311 (1995): 986–89.

Hjemdahl, Paul, MD, PhD 'Stress and the Metabolic Syndrome.' *Circulation* 106, no. 21 (2002): 2634–36.

Jenkins, D. J., et al. 'Nibbling versus Gorging: Metabolic Advantages of Increased Meal Frequency.' *New England Journal of Medicine* 321, no. 14 (1989): 929–34.

Katz, David. *Nutrition in Clinical Practice.* Philadelphia: Lippincott, Williams, and Wilkins, 2001.

Lakka, Hanna-Maaria, MD, PhD 'The Metabolic Syndrome and Total and Cardiovascular Disease Mortality in Middle-aged Men.' *JAMA* 288, no. 21 (2002): 2709–16.

Lawson, O. J., et al. 'The Association of Body Weight, Dietary Intake, and Energy Expenditure with Dietary Restraint and Disinhibition.' *Obesity Research* 3 (1995): 153–61.

Lichtman, S. W., et al. 'Discrepancy between Self-reported and Actual Caloric Intake and Exercise in Obese Subjects.' *New England Journal of Medicine* 327, no. 27 (1992): 1893–98.

Livingstone, M. B. E., et al. 'Accuracy of Weighed Dietary Records in Studies of Diet and Health.' *British Medical Journal* 300 (1990): 708–12.

Ludwig, D. 'Glycemic Index: History and Overview.' *American Journal of Clinical Nutrition* 76 (July 2002): 266S–73S, 267.

Mertz, W., et al. 'What Are People Really Eating?' *American Journal of Clinical Nutrition* 54 (August 1991): 291–95.

Poppitt, S. D., et al. 'Assessment of Selective Underreporting of Food Intake by Both Obese and Nonobese Women in a Metabolic Facility.' *International Journal of Obesity Related Disorders* 22 (1998): 303–11.

Racette, S. B., et al. 'Effects of Aerobic Exercise and Dietary Carbohydrate on Energy Expenditure and Body Composition during Weight Reduction in Obese Women.' *American Journal of Clinical Nutrition* 61 (March 1995): 486–94.

Reaven, G. M. 'Diet and Syndrome X.' *Current Atherosclerosis Reports.* 2, no. 6 (November 2000): 503–7.

Rolls, Barbara J. 'The Role of Energy Density in the Overconsumption of Fat.' *Journal of Nutrition* 130 (2000): 268S–71S.

St Jeor, S. T., et al. 'Dietary Protein and Weight Reduction.' *Circulation* 104, no. 15 (2001): 1869–74.

Samaha, F. F., et al. 'A Low-Carbohydrate as Compared with a Low-Fat Diet in Severe Obesity.' *New England Journal of Medicine* 348, no. 21 (2003): 2074.

Story, M. 'The Prime Time Diet: A Content Analysis of Eating Behavior and Food Messages in Television Program Content and Commercials.' *American Journal of Public Health* 80, no. 6 (1990): 738–40.

Stunkard, A. J., and S. Messick. 'The Three-Factor Eating Questionnaire to Measure Dietary Restraint, Disinhibition, and Hunger.' *Journal of Psychosomatic Research* 29, no. 1 (1985): 71–83.

Stunkard, A. J., et al. 'The Body Mass Index of Twins Who Have Been Reared Apart.' *New England Journal of Medicine* 322, no. 21 (1990): 1483–87.

Wadden, T. A., et al. 'Long-Term Effects of Dieting on Resting Metabolic Rate in Obese Outpatients.' *JAMA* 264, no. 6 (1990): 707–11.

Weinshilboum, R. 'Genomic Medicine.' *New England Journal of Medicine* 348, no. 6 (2003): 529–37.

Whelton, P. K., et al. 'Primary Prevention of Hypertension.' *JAMA* 288, no. 15 (2002): 1882–88.

CREDITS

INDEX

Boldface page references indicate illustrations. <u>Underscored</u> references indicate boxed text.

OTHER RODALE BOOKS
AVAILABLE FROM PAN MACMILLAN

1-4050-2101-2	8 Minutes in the Morning	*Jorge Cruise*	£12.99
1-4050-3284-7	Anti-Ageing Prescriptions	*Dr James A. Duke*	£14.99
1-4050-4099-8	Before the Heart Attacks	*Dr H. Robert Superko*	£12.99
1-4050-4179-X	Fit Not Fat at 40+	*The Editors of* Prevention	£12.99
1-4050-3335-5	Picture Perfect Weight Loss	*Dr Howard Shapiro*	£14.99
1-4050-6717-9	The South Beach Diet Cookbook	*Dr Arthur Agatston*	£20
1-4050-3286-3	Stay Fertile Longer	*Mary Kittel*	£12.99
1-4050-3340-1	When Your Body Gets the Blues	*Marie-Annette Brown and Jo Robinson*	£10.99
1-4050-7330-1	The Women's Health Bible	*The Editors of* Prevention	£14.99

All Pan Macmillan titles can be ordered from our website, *www.panmacmillan.com*, or from your local bookshop and are also available by post from:

Bookpost, PO Box 29, Douglas, Isle of Man IM99 1BQ
Tel: 01624 677237; fax: 01624 670923; e-mail: *bookshop@enterprise.net*; or visit: *www.bookpost.co.uk*. Credit cards accepted. Free postage and packing in the United Kingdom

Prices shown above were correct at time of going to press.

Pan Macmillan reserve the right to show new retail prices on covers which may differ from those previously advertised in the text or elsewhere.

For information about buying *Rodale* titles in **Australia**, contact Pan Macmillan Australia. Tel: 1300 135 113; fax: 1300 135 103; e-mail: *customer.service@macmillan.com.au*; or visit: *www.panmacmillan.com.au*

For information about buying *Rodale* titles in **New Zealand**, contact Macmillan Publishers New Zealand Limited. Tel: (09) 414 0356; fax: (09) 414 0352; e-mail: *lyn@macmillan.co.nz*; or visit: *www.macmillan.co.nz*

For information about buying *Rodale* titles in **South Africa**, contact Pan Macmillan South Africa. Tel: (011) 325 5220; fax: (011) 325 5225; e-mail: *roshni@panmacmillan.co.za*